THE LIVING WELL CODE

10 GUIDING PRINCIPLES TO OPTIMIZE YOUR DAYS & VITALIZE YOUR LIFE

BY DR. TERRY MCCOSKEY AND
LISA NARDELLA MCCOSKEY, CECP

Copyright © 2018 by Terry McCoskey, D.C. &
Lisa McCoskey, CECP

All Rights Reserved.

No part of this publication may be reproduced, distributed, or transmitted in any form or by any means, including photocopying, recording, or other electronic or mechanical methods, or by any information storage and retrieval system without the prior written permission of the publisher, except in the case of very brief quotations embodied in critical reviews and certain other noncommercial uses permitted by copyright law.

Dedication By Lisa McCoskey

I recently realized that book dedications force you to evaluate your relationships and your life. As I was reviewing those thoughts, and all of the wonderful and amazing and motivational people in my life, I felt overwhelmingly thankful and grateful.

My co-author husband, my independent and critical-thinking daughters, and our family of friends have all contributed to this book in one form or another, but the person who has been my guiding influence is my mother, Jean Neary Nardella. Throughout our growing up time, she was consistent in her beliefs about healthy living. She was organic before organic was mainstream. She didn't use aluminum foil, and cooked exclusively in stainless steel. She used tea tree oil, and blackberry brandy for issues and ailments. And thirty years ago, she started her one-woman organic lawn care company called Earth Matters, which is thriving today. Ahead of her time, she is an on-going inspiration in our lives and truly, my mentor.

My dad was the exact opposite. He didn't want to deviate from the tastes and textures of the foods that he enjoyed. Healthier versions of anything were NOT acceptable, and we all knew that. He mastered the art of the dramatic face at the dinner table when something wasn't as it should be - for example, the one-time mom used cottage cheese in lasagna was a culinary Sunday family dinner disaster! Yet, this same man would sit down to a bowl of tripe if it was offered to him.

Interestingly, my dad did embrace chiropractic, but for his whole life, he enjoyed his cold cuts on a hot Italian loaf of bread, spaghetti aioli as a midnight snack, and coffee with no less than 4 heaping teaspoons of sugar. He wasn't a greens eater except for fresh roquette from their garden - grown the way his dad grew it, and his dad before him. We encouraged him to refrain from Coca-cola and cigarettes, but he was a stubborn man. He danced silly dances in the kitchen and loved his family more than life itself. And he liked what he liked and didn't want to give those things up even after his Stage 4 colon cancer diagnosis in April of 2007, which claimed his life 45 days later.

We are each allotted so many days, and we don't know when or how or what will happen to us, but because of my mom's dedication to natural, organic choices, she shaped our lifestyle into a beautiful tapestry of roots, leaves, berries, flowers, sticks, and seeds. She embedded these concepts with a beautiful loving heart, and generously giving hands all because of her desire to do better for her family and for God's planet.

Thank you for sharing your guidance, Mom, and for establishing and maintaining truth in all aspects of our lives. Your wisdom has created a legacy for our children, and our children's children, and our children's children's children.

I love you,

Lisa

DEDICATION BY TERRY MCCOSKEY

There are many people connected to this project. These pages, though, are dedicated to my wife, Lisa, without who's love and support they would not be possible.

Some codes are created for the secret transmission of sensitive information. Others, such as building codes, plumbing codes, and dress codes, are created for rules or laws that must be obeyed. These man-made rules can vary from location to location, and depend on a variety of contingencies.

The Living Well Code is not dependent on man-made regulations, nor is it a necessarily a secret. It has been time-tested and repeated by many of our patients over the last 28 years. These pages are intended to introduce the concepts that we have enjoyed sharing as we watch people reclaim their health and their lives. If you apply them consistently, and share them with friends and family, you will discover the kind of health and vitality your body is naturally designed to possess.

Enjoy!

Table of Contents

- Free Gift For Our Readers 1
- A Note From The Author 2
- Introduction 6
- Principle 1. The Living Well Code 16
- Principle 2. Finding The Intelligence In The Design 23
- Principle 3. Conducting A Symphony 33
- Principle 4. What Goes Up Must Come Down 40
- Principle 5. Fight or Flight 60
- Principle 6. Normal vs. Average vs. Common 70
- Principle 7. He Said, "You Can Eat Anything You Want...Except This." 78
- Principle 8. Visualize yourself: Clothing Optional 122
- Principle 9. Motion is Life 129
- Principle 10. Rest is Restoration 142
- Conclusion 150
- About The Authors 152

Free Gift For Our Readers

As a way of saying "Thank-You" to our readers, we have a special gift for you. Click the link below and you'll have instant access to our Best Self-Guided Imagery video!

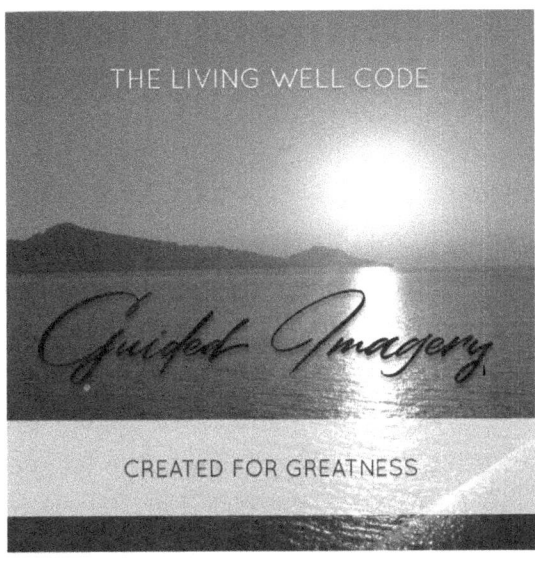

To get your free gift, go to:

https://thelivingwellcode.com/freegift

A Note From The Author

Several years ago, I read an article stating that the average American male lived to 75 years of age. This got me to thinking.

Seventy-five years multiplied by 52 weeks amounts to 3900 weeks. Each week has a Saturday, so this means that the average American male has 3900 Saturdays in his life.

Saturdays are special days. I started picking up my three-year-old grandson for breakfast and errands on Saturday mornings just over three years ago. He can't even remember a time when we didn't do it. He calls it Papaw Day. He is six now and his brother just turned four; sometimes I have one or the other of them, and sometimes I have both boys. It is treasured time for me. If I have only one of them, my wife, Lisa, has the other. That one-on-one time is worth more than gold to both of us.

Usually, unless your work requires you to be there, you'll have Saturdays to do things you'd do rather than working. I wanted a way to consciously make the time count. I wanted to make sure that I was making the most of each day, whether it was for leisure, family time, yard work, golf, or anything else. Time is one of our limitations. None is guaranteed to us, and wasting it is never wise.

At the time I made these calculations of Saturdays, I subtracted the ones I'd already spent. I was 52 at the time, which meant I'd already used 2704 of my Saturdays, and only had 1196 left, assuming I am average. I like to think of myself as above-average, at least in terms of health, but we never know.

I went on Amazon, and ordered 1200 marbles, I keep them in a big glass vase in our dining area. Every Saturday I take a marble out.

This creates a visual reference of time for me. I watch the marbles slowly dwindle. I used to throw them away until one day when my grandson said to me, "Papaw, those are good marbles. Why are you throwing them away?" So we got another vase, and now, every week, he and I transfer one from the bigger to the smaller vase. His brother usually helps, and now it's a ritual we don't miss. We recall the day's adventures and plan for things we'll do in the future. Pure magic.

My hope for you is that after reading this book you realize that each day is a gift. How you spend it may not always be entirely up to you. Life can be hectic and stressful, and not always in your control. But your decisions matter. They have a significant and lasting impact not just on how long, but on how well you live.

You needn't be a millionaire to have a rich and fulfilling life. Your time will eventually expire. But remember, like the dandelion, by casting healthy habits into the world, your life can have a significant impact for generations yet to come.

Preferred Product Link

Throughout the book, we make reference to many personal healthcare products, as well as unique foods and nutrients. We have created a one-stop shop to make it simple and easy for you to find these same items that we recommend to our patients and clients. They have been tested and used by our family, and are organic and/or toxin-free to enhance your overall health and well-being.

Please follow this link to access our preferred products: https://www.amazon.com/shop/alivingwelllife

Introduction

WHY DID WE WRITE THIS BOOK?

You could fill a whole library with books written on the topic of health and wellness. You can find books written from a variety of angles and perspectives, some of which completely contradict each other. There are books on high-fat diets, low-fat diets, and no-fat diets. Some tout a no pain, no gain philosophy. There are books upon books about nutrition, exercise, weight management, and posture. If you can dream of an approach to health and wellness, there is a book about it. Many of these books say exactly the opposite of what the other books say.

So why would I write another book on the topic? What else can be said?

It is exactly this overwhelming amount of contradictory information that compels me to write this book. After spending nearly three decades in the "taking care of people" business, it's become very apparent to me that we don't know the rules for healthy and successful living. America is on the brink of bankruptcy, both economically and energetically. Disease rates are climbing. Young people are now being diagnosed with illnesses typically reserved for the aged. Productivity and happiness are declining. Fear and uncertainty are increasing, while joy and hope for the future are decreasing. The World Health Organization (WHO) currently ranks the US at 37th of the world's industrialized nations.[1]

Nearly twenty cents of every dollar is spent on the management of sickness[2].

Something has to change. This is contrary to the will of God and our essential divine purpose[3].

Health and well-being are not as complicated as those stacks of books would lead us to believe. In my opinion, America doesn't really have a 'health-care crisis.' We just have too many sick people! Pills and potions, bells and whistles in science and technology don't seem to be keeping up with the pace of sickness. In fact, there's an argument to be made that they are quickening the pace.

QUIT BLAMING GENETICS

The human genome hasn't changed since the dawn of time, yet we are being told that genetics are to blame for the increased rate of illness. A lie told often

---

[1] http://www.who.int/whr/2000/media_centre/press_release/en/
[2] https://www.washingtonpost.com/news/wonk/wp/2014/12/03/heres-exactly-how-the-united-states-spends-2-9-trillion-on-health-care/?utm_term=.6c8d32866178
[3] 2 Timothy 1:7 "For God has not given us a spirit of fear, but of power and of love and of a sound mind."

enough is sometimes adopted as truth – is that what is happening?

Let's put some myths to rest and clear up the mystery. The plain and simple truth is that we are managing diseases of lifestyle. The reality is that simple steps, taken consistently and with the intention of living a life free of sickness and disease, will lead you down a path toward Living Well. Living to your full, God-given potential is actually your birthright. In order to realize this birthright, however, you have to learn (and follow) the rules.

You and I have the same genetic code as Moses, Ben Franklin, and every Olympic athlete ever born. It is time to stop blaming our parents for what is wrong with us and take some responsibility for our actions. Psalm 139:14 tells us that we are fearfully and wonderfully made. We are not made with faulty genetics.

The pages that follow are intended to put you back in charge of your life. Your future physical, mental, financial, emotional, and spiritual well-being will depend on your willingness to assume the reins of responsibility for these things. You can't rely upon the government, insurance companies, the pharmaceutical industry, agri-business, or disease management industries to help you. Assuming that they have your best interests at heart is what got us here in the first place. I say "us," because we are all in this together.

Your choices have repercussions that affect everyone, whether or not you understand that this is happening.

It's time to collectively make it right.

HEALTH IS YOUR BIRTHRIGHT

This is intended to be a book of hope. It is intended to help you to understand how the miracle called You has been engineered and programmed for success by a loving Creator. Nothing is random in the design of your body. Each part, from fingernails to liver cells, is dependent on the other parts in some way. We're going to keep it simple, though. Healthy function and healing really are very intricate on a cellular level, but we can explain them in ways that are accessible to everyone. Keeping things simple in this way makes health and hope available to all.

In this book, you will be introduced to concepts, backed by science and supported by Scripture, in a way that allows you to get the "Big Idea" without being overwhelmed by the minutiae of a doctoral level curriculum. We will start at the beginning – in Kindergarten, not graduate school. Starting with the basics and working our way up. Asking the right questions along the way allows for the best kind of learning and effective growth of ideas. You start by reading Dr. Seuss, not Dr. Zhivago – and so we will start our Living Well education the same way.

"There is no greatness where there is not simplicity, goodness, and truth."

– Leo Tolstoy, *War and Peace*

Simple tips and tools that we call "Vitalizers" can be applied consistently to promote or restore normal function. The simplicity, goodness, and truth of these precepts make for the greatness of God's creation. Remember: you are programmed for success, health, joy, recovery, and restoration.

THE DANDELION PRINCIPLE

These 10 Guiding Principles in the Living Well Code will help you repair, restore, and reclaim your health – the physical and mental health that is your birthright.

You will see that making small changes in the choices you make can have far-reaching effects. Think of a dandelion flower in your yard – dandelions have a unique ability to grow anywhere and under almost any condition, whether they are wanted or not. Their life is perpetuated with the slightest breeze – as my yard full of them can attest! You are no different. You are made by the same

Creator. You can make yourself hardy and full of life and further perpetuate this Living Well truth.

I will give you the information you need – and every once in a while, my lovely wife Lisa will give you tips on how to incorporate these guiding principles into your everyday life.

You are fearfully and wonderfully made.

Clarifying Statement:

Some of my early readers informed me that I sounded too harsh, and that telling people genetics were irrelevant was a dangerous idea. The solutions in this book seemed too simple, seemed to ignore psychology and family traits and our upbringings.

I want to make myself clear: as a Doctor of Chiropractic, I work hard to keep current in the science and research regarding health and health care. I have studied the field of epigenetics, not as a geneticist, but as someone who is interested in staying up to date on contemporary science and health. Epigenetics, in a nutshell, is the idea that there are environmental and behavioral factors that will switch a gene on and off. This field of study has completely changed the way health and sickness are viewed.

Certain genes predispose us to certain conditions, but they must be activated by outside stimulus. The proteins that surround each gene must be triggered for that gene to express itself. So, while things like high blood pressure and high cholesterol can run in families, many people with genetic predispositions to those conditions may never express them. People who are born with genetic anomalies like sickle cell anemia or certain heart defects are never going to achieve perfect health on this earth.

Likewise, people sometimes find themselves the victim of circumstances beyond their control. No one asks to be paralyzed as a result of a car accident or fall from a ladder. No one purposefully infects themselves with potentially deadly viruses and bacteria.

I am not talking about these things.

When I speak in this book of your inability to blame genetics and other circumstances for your own fate, I am talking solely about *diseases of lifestyle*. Small children are sometimes unfortunately born with Type I diabetes. This is not a disease of lifestyle. Type II diabetes, brought about by obesity and poor eating habits, however, is a disease of lifestyle.

I recognize that some people are going to work harder to achieve health. My wife talks in this book about her own personal struggle with high blood pressure. Because of her family history, she will have to pay special attention to this issue and work harder than someone who does not have this family history. But still, because she wants to maintain a Living Well Life, she makes the choices she needs to in order to be healthy. And, like a dandelion, the seeds of her example spread to our children and patients and grow beautifully.

I am speaking here only of the choices that you have. This is a personal mission for me. I grew up in a household in which we ate unhealthy foods, and our father smoked. My dad made it to the ripe old Age of 67 and died miserably. Recently, I sadly watched my mom's health disintegrate and then fade away after dementia claimed her life at 74. She could no longer walk or talk, but my heart believes that she knew that I was there for her last breath.

I recognized early on that I needed to make different choices, and my current health reflects that. My brother has the same parents I do, and therefore we resemble each other genetically more than we do any other people on the planet. We come from the same end of the same gene pool. He has, however, made different lifestyle choices and contends with different outcomes as a result of those choices. At only 53 years of age he is currently on medical disability from work due to cardiac insufficiency and Type II Diabetes. We are genetically similar, but our health is vastly different as a result of our choices, not simply because of what we have inherited from our parents.

I have seen too many family members and friends suffer and even die as a result of the choices they make. Of course, I have seen family members and friends suffer and die from things beyond their control, too.

This book attempts to give you the basic information and tools to help you gain the strength to change the things you have the ability to change.

You can enjoy a Living Well life. You can be the best "you" possible. You can live up to your God-given potential. We can't all be supermodels or body builders, some of us will always struggle with poorly functioning kidneys or hearts or misshapen limbs. Getting well takes more effort than staying well. I'm merely suggesting that we have a responsibility to work to reflect the God-given perfection inside of all of us.

DISCLAIMER:

Advice and recommendations given in this book are at the reader's sole discretion and risk. You should see a qualified, licensed doctor before beginning any diet, nutritional, or aromatherapy program. Information presented here is not to be interpreted as an attempt to prescribe or practice medicine. Statements and information in this book have not been evaluated by the Food and Drug Administration. No product offerings or services are intended to treat, diagnose, cure, or prevent any disease. You should always consult a competent, fully-informed medical professional or health practitioner when making decisions for your health. You are advised to investigate and educate yourself about any health-related actions and choices you make.

Principle 1. The Living Well Code

In my 27 years of helping people manage their health, I've noticed a disturbing set of trends. Perhaps you have, too. The information is out there if you know where to look for it.

America is on the brink of a "perfect storm." It's a storm not only of sickness, disease, and death, but economic disaster as well. Consider these facts[4]:

- As of 2012, about half of all adults – that's 11.7 million people! – had one or more chronic health problems.

- 28.4 million adults currently have heart disease, resulting in over 600,000 deaths a year.

- Heart disease and cancer account for 46% of all deaths.

- Obesity affects 36% of all adults – 84 million people!

- Arthritis is the most common cause of disability, affecting 54 million people.

- $3,300,000,000.00 (that's 3.3 TRILLION dollars) was spent in 2016 managing sickness. That's over

---

[4] http://www.cdc.gov/chronicdisease/overview/index.htm

$10,000.00 annually for EVERY man, woman, and child in the US, and 18% of our Gross Domestic Product.

- The leading cause of bankruptcy in the United States is medical expenses[5].

- Chronic illnesses, such as heart disease and diabetes, account for 85% of all health-care costs[6].

- The Kaiser Family Foundation and the Health Research and Educational Trust report that premiums for employer sponsored health insurance in the United States have risen five times faster than workers' earnings since the year 2000.

Life expectancy is the average number of years a child born today would live if current mortality patterns remain the same. In a pre-modern, poor world, life expectancy was around 30 years in all regions of the world. In the early 19th century, life expectancy began to increase in the early industrialized countries while it stayed low in the rest of the world.

Since 1900, the global average life expectancy has more than doubled and is now approaching 70 years. To what are these increases attributed? Scientists suggest

---

[5] http://www.investopedia.com/financial-edge/0310/top-5-reasons-people-go-bankrupt.aspx
[6] http://www.thebalance.com/causes-of-rising-healthcare-costs-4064878

three main causes: knowledge, science, and technology[7]. "Directly through the application of new ideas about personal health and public administration, and indirectly through increased productivity that permitted (albeit with some terrible reversals) better levels of living, better nutrition, better housing, and better sanitation.[8]"

In other words, once we got the hang of not consuming the same water in which we bathe and remove our waste, things began to improve significantly.

But is living longer the same as living better? That depends on who you ask. There is an argument to be made for allowing lives to expire without the heroics of modern technology. Keeping people 'alive' is very different that allowing people to have a fulfilling and vital experience on the planet.

On the opposite side, technology may create reversals in certain conditions, thereby promoting longevity; this additional time can prove a blessing to many. This book is not the place for the moral and ethical debate or the policies and politics that can cloud this issue. Rather, I'll simply encourage our readers to focus

---

[7] David Cudler, Angus Deaton, and Adriana Lleras-Muney (2006) "The Determinants of Mortality." Journal of Economic Perspectives, 20(3) 97-120.
[8] Id.

on the things they can do to maintain the quality of life they desire.

By anyone's definition, this would have to be considered a crisis situation. The question becomes: how long can this possibly be sustainable?

From the outset, let me suggest that we don't necessarily have a 'health-care crisis.' What we do have, however, is far too many sick people. Rather than attempting to constantly resolve a nationwide 'crisis,' I'll suggest that we simply begin to focus on decreasing the number of sick people. The pages that follow contain my suggestions for making this happen: a code of conduct, if you will, a Living Well Code. Our goal is to provide a solution to this problem.

While some codes are developed to hide or encrypt sensitive information, this is exactly the opposite. This is more along the lines of the rules or laws, such as building codes, plumbing codes, or dress codes, that must be obeyed to ensure that everyone is safe and comfortable. These man-made rules can vary from place to place, and depend on a variety of contingencies.

The Living Well Code is different, in that it is not dependent on man-made regulations or cultural norms. It may well be the world's best kept secret, though. It has been time tested and repeated successfully by many of our patients over the last 27 years. You will read some of their stories in the pages to come.

This book is intended to introduce the concepts we have enjoyed sharing as we watch people reclaim their health and their lives. If you apply them consistently, and share them with family and friends, you can find the kind of health and vitality your body is naturally designed to express.

The sooner you begin to make the changes we discuss, the sooner you become part of the solution. Our promise to you is the results! While change is never as easy as we'd like, starting today is what moves you toward a happier and healthier life. All you have to do is keep reading and apply what you learn in each chapter. Sharing what you learn can be contagious, too. Lisa and I look forward to assisting you on your journey to a better life.

VITALIZERS:

1. Be aware of the information around you. Stay abreast of the latest health news and always seek its source.

2. Change doesn't happen overnight. Stick with it, and you WILL see results!

Note from Lisa:

Throughout the years, Terry and I have witnessed miracles: awe-inspiring and life-changing miracles.

The highlights of my day include reports back from clients, friends, and family members who have applied a personalized protocol or simply safe-swapped a laundry detergent or make-up foundation to toxin-free, and are now living a better life as a result. They have eliminated hot flashes and acid reflux, lost weight that's been stuck for years, and finally enjoyed a deep restorative night's sleep, with a joyful mood in the morning.

Knowing that the ripple effect from these changes creates happier partnerships and parenting, which creates motivated employees and focused students, which creates thankful employers and teachers which generates abundance within communities - reaching farther beyond what we can ever know - is humbling. All beginning from one better choice and the awareness that we are each created to help and serve others in the capacity that we were designed for the good of His Kingdom.

This inspired action, this message of health and vitality paired with the Word of God, provides hope in a world where it is desperately needed. I've seen these applied principles manifest the extraordinary from the ordinary and transform lives in magnificent ways, and I am excited to see you transform yours as well!

Thank you for taking this journey with us. I'm sure you'll be glad you did.

Principle 2. Finding The Intelligence In The Design

Destruction is not Construction

Regardless of how you or others think the universe got here, I think we can all agree that the universe is a pretty smart place. I have heard it said by educated people that the universe formed billions of years ago as a result of a rather big bang. Here is my big bang story:

As a much younger person, my friends and I thought it would be interesting to replicate army adventures from movies and TV. The idea was to take our GI Joe action figures, secure them in their cool plastic Jeeps, and strap on some M80s with tape. We'd light the fuses and speed them down the driveway, cheering the chaos created by the bang the firecrackers made. We would repeat the challenge with metal Tonka trucks and structures made of Popsicle sticks and the results were nothing short of awesome. My parents, naturally, were unimpressed.

My experience revealed that explosions, even relatively small ones, tend to disorganize things. I just cannot comprehend how many millions of years it would take for Joe and his Jeep to return, re-organized, to their original splendor. The fact that they are buried in a landfill in southeastern Ohio makes it somehow even more difficult to imagine. It's only been forty or so years ago, so I doubt they've had sufficient time yet.

What I know is this: GI Joe and his Jeep didn't suddenly spring into being. Someone had to think up the idea of GI Joe. Then they had to act with intent on that thought by sketching it and making a prototype.

The prototype was then pitched to a company so they could further the idea. Once the idea was accepted, then there were product designers, engineers, plastics makers, focus groups, production line employees, and so on.

They did not design GI Joe and then accidentally end up with Barbie or Ken. Each one was designed separately through a similar, but not identical, process. Joe, as incredible as he was prior to our little experiment, did not manifest from a molecular mishap in the universe millions of years ago.

And neither did you.

Time wears things down. Things erode and decompose. The large explosion theory as a method of creation is a stretch my mind just can't make. Over time, things become less organized, not more. Think of composting – vegetation returns to its essential elements; it doesn't turn into something new. Think of having to repaint your house every few years because the paint breaks down. There had to have been intention, design, a designer, a builder, and a plan involved in your creation. There's intelligence at work, and you're a part of it. The evidence is overwhelming.

"Before I formed you in the womb I knew you; Before you were born, I set you apart."

Jeremiah 1:5

SOME THINGS TO PONDER:

- How do birds know which way is south for the winter?
- Are seeds alive or dead?
- What is it that allows an apple seed to turn into an apple tree?
- How can a sperm from a male combine with an egg from a female of the same species and, under just the right conditions and at just the right time, produce an entirely new and similar, but distinctly different offspring?

MIRACLES ARE EVERYWHERE

I think we have been so bombarded with the latest and greatest gadgets and gizmos that we have been desensitized to the common miracles of life. If I am allowed to spend my free time, in unlimited amounts, in front of a glowing screen of photo-shopped fictional images, I may very well miss the things in the natural world that reveal how incredibly remarkable and intelligent this place is. Sure, the occasional bird gets lost or confused, but the overwhelming majority seem to make it to bask in the warmer climates and watch the human 'snowbirds' play golf and walk the beaches.

Conditions matter. This intelligence does not simply create, out of thin air, at random moments. There are limitations. Not every seed becomes the majesty of a tree. Some suffer the effects of drought; some never make it to fertile soil. Still others are picked up as food by something higher up in the food chain.

THERE IS NO LAW GREATER THAN NATURAL LAW

Speaking of the food chain: have you ever noticed that animals seem to eat only the things that nourish them? Some eat only meat; some eat only vegetables. But have you ever heard elephants in the wild with acid reflux or allergies? They never seem as confused as we do about such things.

Certain plants and animals are specific to certain regions. Every time we try to transplant them, chaos ensues. Take kudzu, for example. Native to Japan, it was brought to the American south and used as a food for livestock and as erosion control. Now, this invasive species which can grow up to a foot a day is strangling and uprooting native trees. Fighting the creep of kudzu is difficult and an industry in and of itself. This chaos and destruction is entirely the result of humans interfering with the natural law.

There are processes in nature that are most beneficial for the overall good of the order. Plant growth; forestation (and deforestation with natural wildfire); the establishment of wetlands and deserts; fresh water and salt water generation; and the perpetuation of a species – all of these things seem to require more time, energy, and resources than the events that can destroy them.

How long does it take to grow a forest? But how long does it take to burn it down? And what happens once the fire is out? That's right – regeneration of a living, organized ecosystem. Automatically. The Gulf of Mexico began recovering even before the man-made oil spill had been capped. But, unlike a mythical phoenix rising from the ashes, devastation comes quickly, and recovery takes more time. Always.

The Intelligence of the systems that are in place simply requires what it requires, including time. There is no way to change this. Natural laws have no regard for us and our desires, our social status, our bank account, or anything else. Imagine planting your garden today and expecting fresh vegetables tomorrow. Not realistic, right? So why do we expect unrealistic things all the time? When it comes to health and healing, we want it yesterday. How long does it take to grow a healthy femur? Years! How long to break it? A split second. How long does it take to heal? Weeks or even months – if ever. Burns, cuts, abrasions, colds, flu, cancer, arthritis, heart disease all take time to heal. We'll think of dozens, maybe hundreds, of ways to outsmart the system.

But over-riding the Intelligence comes with a price.

VITALIZERS:

1. Recognize the intelligence in your design on a daily basis. And take a moment to be thankful.
2. Good health is your divine birthright – assume that it is achievable for you.
3. Make sure you act in accordance with natural law (your intelligent design.) If you fail to do so, it comes with a price. Actions & consequences.

NOTES FROM LISA:

A long, long time ago, when I was 12 or 13, I read a book called *A Tree Grows in Brooklyn* by Betty Smith. The book was first published in 1945, but its message is timeless.

It was a book that evoked an extremely emotional response in my young life. It opened my eyes to how blessed I was to have a family, immediate and extended, and a Heavenly Father that loved me, unconditionally. I hadn't known there was any other way, and it created compassion and thankfulness and appreciation in my heart.

The title of the book comes from a part of the story that refers to a young sapling tree that had pushed its way through the cracks in the sidewalk of Francie's, the main character's, neighborhood. This image is a symbol of how, even in the most adverse circumstances, we are created to survive.

Nasturtiums, are experts at that, and they always remind me of that revelational time in my life when I learned that we were created to persevere, survive, and, even more than that, to blossom in a beautiful, compassionate, and thankful way as voices for God and servants of His Kingdom. I spotted this flower on my way to lunch with my precious daughters, and felt overwhelmed by God's loving promises to me as I revisited that time in my life.

Like you, I have spent too much time in my life being overwhelmed by life's journey instead of God's love. Haven't you ever just wanted to crawl under your covers and sleep forever? Has your to-do list ever threatened to swallow you alive? Are you having difficulty finding peace in any corner of your life?

Admittedly, this is me. Right here, right now. Sometimes I lose focus of God's love and the blessings in my life.

My morning ritual centers around time spent with God. Sometimes I am fully engaged, sometimes I am going through the motions. Today, my Heavenly Father wrapped me in his loving arms and gently spoke into my heart.

The conversation went like this:

"God? God? Where are you?"

"I am here, Lisa. I am always here."

"I don't feel you and I'm scared."

"Fear is not of me. I see you, and I see your struggles, and I know your heart."

"Life feels out of control. I am out of control. I fear that I am not serving you or the Kingdom the way You intended, and that my focus flits away from You in an instant. I need to know You're near."

"I will never leave you nor forsake you. You know that. You study that. You share that."

"I feel like that's a cliché. Am I too far ahead of You? Too far behind?"

"I am walking with you. You also know that."

"I'm not sure I do."

silence

Then, he whispered, *"Mind your mind."*

tears

Sometimes, we just need simple truth. And then we must take control of what we are given control over. Period. We have dominion over our thoughts and we can purposely release fear, anxiety, and negative self-talk. "I'm not good enough." "I'll never get this done." "I am not equipped." "I'm running out of time." "Another mistake." "Can't you remember anything anymore?" These are taunting sentences and lies from the enemy. Every single one of them.

There's still work to be done here. My mission for Him is not complete. So today, I am taking back my mind, and redirecting my focus. I know that by writing this, I become a larger target. But I also know Who provides my armor, so I'm vitalizing my life by:

- Releasing all "Shoulds," "Oughts," and "Haves."

- Speaking to myself the way I speak to others.

- Affirming my place in the Kingdom by repeating, "I was made and created by the God of the Bible.[9] I am fully equipped by Him and for Him. I am loved and beloved. And I am saved by the blood of Jesus Christ."

My hope is that by sharing this personal story that you will vitalize yourself, put on the armor of God, and mind your mind.

This is the day that God has made. Let's rejoice in that together!

---

[9] https://www.bible.com/bible/1/PSA.83.kjv

Principle 3. Conducting A Symphony

I love music. I am not a musician, but I deeply appreciate the gifts and talents of others who can take something as simple as a few strings stretched over a hollow object and make it do magical things. Blues, jazz, classical, bluegrass, funk, Native American, cultural, and ethnic music all tell stories. Music, given the right genre in the right situation, can set a tone or mood that enhances any experience. Imagine the Lion King, Rock, or even Sesame Street without music.

THE SONG OF YOUR LIFE

Let's take a look at you. The song of your life tells a story. Your opening notes were a single microscopic cell from your father and a single microscopic cell from your mother. Under just the right circumstances and just the right conditions, at just the right time, those opening notes became the symphony that is you: the person listed on your birth certificate. Not the person you see in the mirror today – we'll get to that person later. But before you were You, two simple cells multiplied and divided and differentiated in very well synchronized and symphonic ways.

Consider this: a concert "G" has unlimited potential, it can begin something as complicated and wondrous as Beethoven's iconic Fifth Symphony or as simple as "Row Row Row Your Boat." The difference is not in the "G" but in the act of the composer and the musician – your wondrous being is no different. The Intelligent Creator (God) and the Musician (You) have worked together to create your song.

Certain things had to happen in a certain order. Just like the "G" has to be followed by an "E-flat" in order to begin Beethoven's Symphony, your heart cells, skin cells, or liver cells could not develop before nerve cells. In fact, nothing could develop before nerve cells. The Conductor of this masterpiece called You first differentiates the cells of the nervous system from the undifferentiated stem cells. Their task is to control and direct the development of the rest of the organism. Their job doesn't end with the signing of your birth certificate. They remain at the top – in your brain – to be the Conductor of all cellular function throughout life. They are in charge of sight, sound, taste, touch, and smell. They are the rulers over emotion, creativity, hormone balance, muscle movement. Everything you sense, do, and experience is sensed, done, and experienced through your master nervous system. What a job!

Clean, clear signals in the messages sent from the brain to the body are essential to keep you alive in this moment. These nerve cells are so important that the hardware, your brain and spinal cord, are encased in protective bone. The skull and spinal column are literally a protective conduit and breaker box for the vital impulses that travel this system and animate you.

Think of it this way: When are people pronounced dead? Not when their heart stops – we just try to restart it. Not when their kidney functions cease – that's what dialysis is for. These things can even be replaced or transplanted if need be. It is the flat line on the monitor that represents the lack of functional brain signal that marks the end of life. Brain dead is dead.

I say this to set the stage for the rest of this book. If you're one of those people that glosses through a book by skipping from chapter to chapter, you may miss this critical nugget. If you do, it's over, and none of the rest of it will make any sense.

The body you are living in functions on one major premise: Homeostasis.

Homeostasis, according to dictionary.com, is "the tendency of a system, especially the physiological system of higher animals, to maintain internal stability, owing to the coordinated response of its parts to any situation or stimulus that would tend to disturb its normal condition or functions."

What that means is that, like water will always seek its own level, your body is always seeking to find its level best. It is designed to resist changes to the basic operating system. That resistance takes the shape of aches, pains and disease.

In any given moment while you are alive, the primary role of the nervous system is in the maintenance of homeostasis. Simply put, that means detecting changes in the environment and input, and providing the things necessary for the cells of the body to function in harmony.

When it is cold, you shiver to produce warmth. When there is a lot of light, your pupils constrict to prevent blindness. Millions of bits of information result in changes that are designed to keep you alive.

Too much or too little of anything upsets this delicate balance. This is true even if it is a good thing. We know that we should exercise and eat fresh fruit. But too much exercise can result in damage to joints or bones. Too much organic fruit can result in digestive troubles. Too much or too little of whatever substance or activity can result in toxicity or a deficiency in the equilibrium of your body. Once the delicate balance is upset, it results in a series of changes that begin to affect the health of the organism called You.

It's All About the Nervous System

It seems that everyone in 'authority' in our healthcare delivery system seems quite willing to overlook this little detail. Doctors of Chiropractic (D.C.s) are the only ones in the healing arts focused on this seemingly simple fact: everything mentioned from here forward must be in the context of understanding the supremacy of the Creator's intent for the nervous system.

The Intelligence that formed you from two disconnected cells did not abandon you at birth. Its role in the regulation of all life function cannot be overstated. Any health and wellness program that does not include caring for the nervous system and the spine that houses it cannot be a complete system and is destined to fail. Chiropractic doctors are the only providers in today's healthcare system trained to recognize the supremacy of the nervous system.

Does this sound like a bold statement? Well, acknowledging the intelligence inherent in all living things requires a certain degree of boldness. Acknowledging a loving Creator in the scientific process seems difficult for some as well. Fixing a health care system that's out of control will also require some powerful determination. Good luck – You're fully equipped!

―――――――――――――

Vitalizers:

1. When something in the song of your life is 'out of tune,' see a Chiropractor. They are the only

medical professionals that will tune your instrument at its source.

2. Trust your body. It's smarter than you.

3. Restoring homeostasis is like tuning the symphony of your life. It is the key to restoring healthy function.

Notes from Lisa:

Music has always been a part of my life. My amazingly multi-talented mother is a skilled pianist. I loved sitting next to her, on the piano bench in front of her baby grand, when we were growing up, and watching her fingers adeptly hit the exact right notes at the exact right time, while my sister and brother and I would sing along. My dad would be nearby watching this musical scene unfold usually with the Red Sox game on, but sometimes he would participate in the singing by making up his own words, or if he had a special request like, "Jean" by Johnny Mathis. My mom's name is Jean and my dad was a romantic man, so he would sing dramatically, but lovingly, to her as she played. We would all laugh with him, and then he'd go back to watching the game.

I still remember the music book with its golden decorative binding; but to truly be of service to my mom on that piano bench, I needed to know when to turn the pages in the book. I needed to know how to read the music so I could follow along and get it right. Musical notes are mysterious, but like punctuation, those marks create a story. Mom took the time to teach each of us how to unravel the mystery of those notes - to simplify what seemed so complex. She explained the count for each type, and the tune for each line that the note was attached to. She gently explained rhythm, pitch and tone, and the nuances of the dots and dashes throughout the scores. When played correctly it became a succession of notes, that was pleasing to the ear.

And then when I was in the 7th grade, the band instructor recommended that I learn to play the saxophone. That sounded intriguing and my parents bravely agreed to it. The process was overwhelming at first, but what I realized was that those notes I had learned to play on the piano were the same notes that I followed to play the saxophone, because music is a universal language similar to the universal language of living well. When the rules of the language are recognized, understood and followed, there is harmony and beauty in the creation, but when the rules are broken, altered, or ignored, then chaos and cacophony ensue.

Thankfully, God's only request about music is to worship with a joyful noise, and I think we accomplished that; even our dog, Ginger, seemed to enjoy the commotion. But He also instructs us to respect our bodies as Holy Temples, to remember that we are to treat them with the honor that they deserve knowing Who created them. This requires from us a willingness and a desire to follow God's guidebook for living well.

Principle 4. What Goes Up Must Come Down

GRAVITY

Nothing would seem heavy if it weren't for gravity. It's a force that is constant and that holds everything on the planet. It's the reason that "what goes up, must come down." Sir Isaac Newton discovered the theory of gravity, and was able to use advanced mathematics to understand how it works.

Newton is most famous for discovering the law of gravity, but he also discovered several other laws of physics that are part of our immutable universe. He determined that every action must have an equal but opposite reaction. He stated that a body at rest tends to stay at rest, unless acted upon by an outside force. We will talk more on this later when we talk about movement and exercise.

Before we go any further, I'd like to address some questions you may have. Newton is considered the father of modern mathematics and science. Conventional wisdom holds that his ideas are the basis of the big bang theory and other theories that deny the existence of an intelligent Creator. How then, you may be asking, can I uphold His theories as well as that of intelligent design?

What most people forget – or what they never learned, because they were never taught in school, is that Newton himself was a strong proponent of intelligent design. In his seminal work Mathematica Principia, written in 1686, he said, "This most beautiful system of the sun, planets, and comets, could only proceed from the counsel and dominion of an intelligent and powerful Being. This Being governs all things, not as the soul of the world, but as Lord over all, and an account of His dominion He is wont to be called Lord God, Universal Ruler." Clearly Newton himself did not think his ideas and mathematics in conflict with the existence of a Creator. So why should we?

If this sounds like cherry-picking, understand this: most of science is cherry-picking. Place holders like "dark matter" account for what science cannot explain. The denial of a Creator or Designer eliminates many absolutes, including moral absolutes. This paves the way for destructive behavior, for a collective "if it feels good, do it" culture. We're there, and we are reaping the results.

THE ENGINEERING OF YOUR BODY

While you are engineered to function in this Earthly environment, there's always a price to be paid when the laws of nature are ignored.

Just as the components of a building are placed just so – an I-beam here, a rivet there, bricks stacked in a particular pattern – so are the components of your body. Posture does matter. All structures, man-made and natural, are engineered to be in a specific place and a particular order if they are to withstand outside forces and not collapse in on themselves.

So, what is the properly engineered structure of the human body? Within certain boundaries, a 10-12-pound head should be centered over a balanced neck and a set of level shoulders. Level shoulders should be balanced over a set of level hips. Level hips result in level leg length and an even distribution of a body versus gravity. In other words, if you weighed 100 pounds, how much weight should be balanced on each foot? 50 pounds, of course.

"But wait a minute," you may say. "I thought everyone had one leg shorter than the other."

Remember, there's a difference between something that is common and something that is normal – normal here being defined as "as it should be" or "according to plan." Abnormal body alignment is common and starts to leave clues. If your shirt or tie drift to one side, or your necklace hangs off-center, or if one pant leg drags on the ground when you walk, that's a big clue that your body isn't in normal alignment. If one hip or knee begins to wear out ahead of the other, that's another clue. One shoe may wear out before the other. These are all clues that you should seek help.

Sometimes in a chiropractic or orthopedic office you'll hear the phrase "bone on bone." This means that one set of joints has been out of balance for such an extended period of time that the cartilage cushions between them have worn away. You may ignore the clues you have been given – so you have to buy new shoes more often, or constantly straighten your necklace. Who cares? Well, it is easier to get new shoes than new joints. Don't ignore these obvious clues.

Unfortunately, when spinal injury or damage occurs, at any age, the muscles and ligaments that support the body in this balanced position begin to fail. This process of degenerative wear and tear is accelerated to an inflammatory nightmare called osteoarthritis. But the mechanical decay and its accompanying discomfort are only part of the equation. If the delicate nerves that transmit information to and from the brain are compromised, the health of the organism can be challenged in many ways. This clinical phenomenon is known as Vertebral Subluxation. Body chemistry can be compromised. What if the nerves to the heart are affected? Or the pancreas? Or the adrenal glands? Now we have a bigger problem that may not have obvious symptoms for quite some time. All of these secondary conditions will likely have a spinal connection as the nerves that exit as specific spinal levels affect the performance of those organs.

Limitations

In science, matter is the term for any type of material. 'Matter' is anything that has mass and takes up space.

I can't think of anything of a physical nature that doesn't have limits. Cars can only go so fast. Metal will only bend so far without breaking. The mightiest oak trees will succumb to fire or wind when their limits are exceeded. Even light has a speed limit. Your body is no different.

While your mind can expand to amazing extremes, your physical body cannot. It has limitations that cannot be exceeded. I believe these limitations were placed within each of us for certain purposes, one of which is to let us know we are not God. He has no limitations. We, as humans, do.

Another purpose for these limitations is so that we can learn to rely on the strengths and gifts of others as we figure out how to get along. There are limits of strength and stamina that are similar among us, but clearly different for some.

For example, as a younger person, I covered a 100-yard dash in under 11 seconds. I did a 220-yard dash in under 23 seconds, and a quarter mile right around 51 seconds. My long jump was just over 20 feet. I was not exactly Olympic material, but I was above average and better than most of my peers at the time. Today, no way! I believe those are what are referred to as "The Glory Days." Predictably, my limits have changed with time.

Even if I were to prioritize my training again, I still doubt the likelihood of achieving those marks as a more "seasoned citizen." Some limits are self-imposed, but others are not.

I've heard the expression, "If you can believe it, you can achieve it." While this phrase has some merit, it is never going to be entirely true. No matter how hard I believe I can, I will never be able to long jump 40 feet, for example. I'll never win the Tour de France, even though my mind can easily visualize myself crossing the Champs-Elysees, hands raised in victory. The likelihood of seeing me on television accepting the coveted green jacket from having won the Masters Golf Tournament is also pretty slim.

Limits are for a purpose. If your physical body has been injured or compromised beyond its limitations for full functions, you may not be able to do some of the things we will talk about in the pages that follow. If you've been afflicted with a disease process beyond your genetic capacity for 100% function, you may have to modify these recommendations to suit your reality. That's okay! As we acknowledge our limitations, let's always remember their purposes and work hard to maximize our potential within those limits.

Knowing that we, as humans, are a special creation, different from the other animals on the planet, able to write music and construct skyscrapers, let's focus on appreciating our limits as we strive to live up to the expectations set for us by our creator.

Can limits change? Some can, some can't.

Modifying limitations is a function of adaptability, If I could do five pushups and then rested, I could do five more. Then ten. I could actually improve my initial limit if I continued to strive to do so. Could I reach fifty or seventy-five? Maybe, but there will be a point at which I achieve a maximum limit.

The limitations of my discipline will be tested, too. I'm not sure the actual number is the most important lesson here. Who I become in reaching that number is likely more important than the number itself. Be disciplined. Be determined. Be unwilling to settle for less than your best. These are good qualities for living your best life.

The Spine as Breaker Box

Think of it like the breaker box in your home. Power comes into the house from the outside. The breaker box is designed for two things: One, the distribution of power to various locations for light, heat, cooling, and other things you need electricity for. Two, protection from an overload of electricity. Without protection from overload, your entire electrical system can be damaged, and the likelihood of fire goes up substantially.

Some of us are 'mature' enough to remember the days of a fuse box. Too much electricity would result in burning out a fuse, which could then be replaced. If you didn't have any fuses on hand, you could jerry-rig an electrical connection by wedging a penny in the slot to complete the circuit and restore power. Unfortunately, simply replacing the fuse (or reconnecting the circuit) without determining the cause of the overload could result in more electrical surges, which could result in fire. Thus, the development of the modern circuit breaker system which is designed to flip a switch before things get out of hand. Smarter. Safer.

Your spine is the breaker box for your body. It allows for the distribution of normal nerve signals to govern all life function and is designed to give you signals when the load limit has been exceeded. The signal might be pain, but it might be something else as well. The

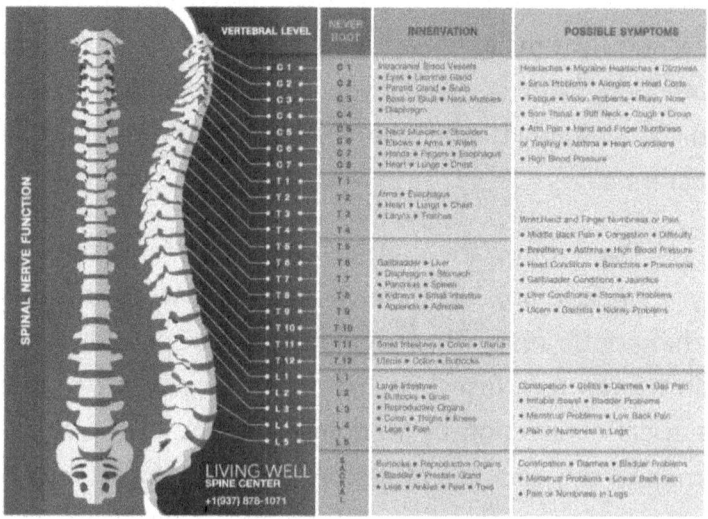

resulting imbalance could be increased signals to different parts of your body that result in overload and malfunction. Is your stomach acid too high or too low? What signal is your stomach getting, and how clear is that signal? Is your heart running too fast or too slow? What signal is your brain transmitting to your heart?

How do you know what these signals are and what they mean? Start by simply following the nerves back to the breaker box panel that is your spine to begin solving the mystery. Pain is never the problem in and of itself. It is just a signal that says 'check me,' just like the engine light in your car or a flipped breaker in your electrical system. Taking pain relievers doesn't solve any problems – it is no different than the penny jammed into the fuse box of old. It doesn't address the reason for the overload. The result of ignoring the source of the signal can be a metaphorical house fire for your health.

The most common complaint we've seen in our office over the years is pain. Headaches, spinal pain, and joint pain are what drive most people to seek our help. Initially, anyway.

Upon further investigation, people find that it's easy to connect the dots between their other health concerns and relief through chiropractic care. Why would a 'spine doctor' be concerned enough to ask about constipation, indigestion, irritable bowel, paresthesia, infertility, chronic infections, cardiovascular issues, or any other symptoms beyond basic pain? It's simple.

These issues are all connected to the same brain that moves the muscles that lock the joints that causes the pain. We can explore the 'breaker box' of our spine and follow the 'wires,' or nerves, back to their source using surface electromyography (SEMG.) When we do this, understanding the malfunctions becomes easy. It's common to find abnormal nerve signals that can only result in abnormal function.

You can see a 3D visual of this by clicking on this link:

https://mymisalignment.com/livingwellspinecenter

The location of apparent symptoms and their point of origin often do not match. A pain in your hand may not mean an injury to your hand. Again, the circuit breaker analogy works well. If you are blow drying your hair with the exhaust fan, a curling iron, and a radio turned on, you may overload the bathroom circuits. This results in a blown fuse in the basement circuit breaker box, which then in turn results in a darkened living room. Pain and muscle spasms are the result of your body's fuse being blown, which is a signal to you that homeostasis has been interrupted.

It's very common to see a multitude of other conditions get resolved with corrective spinal care. Your body is always seeking to restore itself. It does a better job of restoration when all the circuits are open and functioning as they should.

JOHN'S STORY

John came to us originally because of neck pain. He'd suffered with it for years. He developed migraine headaches that were so severe he missed work frequently.

As the owner of his own business, this was disastrous: no work = no income.

Within a matter of weeks after coming to see us, John's migraines and pain had all but stopped. He was thrilled with this outcome, but wanted to take it a step further. He said, "Could this have anything to do with my bowels?"

"Why do you ask?" I responded.

His answer was tearful. "I've had such irritable bowels for the last several years that leaving the house was all but impossible. I kept spare underwear at work, in my car, my wife's car, and her purse. It was horribly embarrassing. But it stopped! I'm having normal movements and control that I never expected to see again. I've been on every imaginable drug and had no results. It's a miracle!

"Another issue has been the anxiety and cardiac distress connected to these things! My heart sometimes felt like it would race out of my chest. It's gone!"

The miracle, of course, is not in the cure, but in the creation of the system itself. John's body was designed to function in a certain way. When his 'breaker box' was not allowing the proper signals to flow the way they should, everything got out of whack. When we restored normal spinal and nerve function, many of his other secondary issues began to resolve as well!

Here's a more personal example of a time in which a lot of my limits were tested and how I could see, first hand, what happened when the breaker box was not allowed to send its signals properly.

When our daughter was in her 20th hour of labor with our first grandson, it became obvious that she would be having a C-section. The limitations of matter had been reached in her body and in the baby's body.

The surgery went well, and our grandson was delivered. The new Mom was sent to recovery with Lisa. Our son-in-law was off to the Neonatal Intensive Care Unit (NICU) with Hawk, our new boy. Hawk was placed in the NICU because his respiratory rate was twice the expected for a newborn. He looked perfect from the outside, but the monitors were telling a different story on the inside. The doctors wanted to keep an eye on him to calculate their next move.

The new Pawpaw, me, was in Ohio while this was happening in Georgia. I awaited the green light to head south. Twenty-seven hours would pass before I got to lay eyes on him. Distance, traffic, and time made a stressful situation worse.

Upon arrival, everyone involved was exhausted and I was made aware that visiting hours were over. Thankfully, the nurse in the NICU had some mercy and allowed the new daddy and me to have five minutes with Hawk.

He was a handsome little man, lying there all bundled up under the warmer. My heart was forever changed when I saw him. My child's child. Perfect. Except the monitors didn't agree with what appeared at first glance. His heart rate, oxygen saturation, respiratory rate, temperature, and blood pressure were all being monitored on a screen in front of us and indicated something was modifying his homeostatic balance. Let's face it – he'd just been through a rough start! He was stressed, and his autonomic system was in overdrive.

Interestingly, his little head was tilted significantly towards his left shoulder, which certainly couldn't be comfortable. I knew that posture matters, and that these muscles would have some work to do before he would have control of his head. I also knew that his body would always be seeking to do the right thing. I simply moved his head to its center over his shoulders.

He didn't mind at all, but the monitors certainly took note! Within seconds, all of his numbers moved towards normal. His respiratory rate in particular began to settle as I held his head in neutral. I took my hand away and his head drifted back over his left shoulder. All of the numbers began to rise again. Cause and effect? You decide.

After stabilizing his head in a better place with a light touch to the neck, we again watched his numbers settle down. My son-in-law and I had a nice cry, and we all settled in to get some rest.

The next morning in the NICU, Hawk's numbers were better, but still not good enough for him to be released. I gave him another light touch and got another favorable response in return. Homeostasis was on its way.

We later learned that the average stay in the NICU is 12-14 days with this challenge. Treatment could range from breathing treatments to a variety of other drugs.

We were leaving with a happy, healthy boy on the third day. He was given no drugs or other interventions.

Vitalizers:

1. Seek first to find the cause of symptoms rather than to alter them with chemistry.

2. A proper Chiropractic spinal health evaluation is a safe and conservative way to assess your structural alignment and the integrity of your nervous

system. Body alignment is a signal that the structure is intact.

NOTES FROM LISA:

Chicken, dolphin trainer, cheerleader, horseback rider, jewelry designer, "silly whim", artist, dancer, mommy, dog, jewelry maker, song writer: this is just a short list of some of the "careers" our daughters wanted to be when they grew up.

When we're young, the world is full of limitless possibilities that are explored daily through stories and imagination! It seems real to us that if we want to be a dog, we can be a dog. It is no different than wanting to be a teacher or an astronaut. Every day is a new adventure and we think about the ideas that are thrilling to us! We dream BIG!!

My husband has known since he was in the 7th grade that he would be a chiropractor. Not everyone has the advantage and privilege of knowing what their career will be that early on in life, but it was a true calling and every one of the gifts that he possesses is suited to this profession. He is a doctor and teacher, and has the communication skills to effectively reach tens of thousands of people a year, helping them understand the connection between their spine, their nervous system, and their lives. He is a master of the analogy, explaining spinal care to each unique person in the language they understand. Whether they are engineers, mechanics, homemakers, CEO's, or athletes, he can equate what he does to what they already know. It is a true gift! As his wife, I reap the benefit of his joy, his elation over God's miracles as he witnesses them every single day, especially when they are miracles for one's very own grandson.

Twenty-eight years ago, being a chiropractor's wife brought a lot of questioning glances, and some careless and uninformed comments. We lived life differently than most. Well-baby visits consisted of a maintenance schedule for upper cervical chiropractic care from the time our daughters were born. We had food from the one health food store on the other side of town. We had an herb cabinet, instead of a medicine chest, and one designated for tea. We birthed our babies at home. We chose not to vaccinate. We churched at home, and then when we began homeschooling our daughters, many friends, some family, and random community members, could not understand why we would ever take on that alleged burden. They would ask "why would you do that?", "what about socialization", "isn't our system good enough?", "are you even qualified?", "how long will you be able to keep this up?".

As a young mother, new to maternal things, I was not yet immune to the stinging criticism. Initially, it was offensive to me, and I was thankful for a solid foundation from which our decisions were made, but I needed a response - a sweet, soft, honey response - to diffuse the questioning. I found that by simply stating, "It might not work for everyone, but this works for us," was enough to end the discussion.

That answer allowed me to take a non-defensive stance. I was not going to get into a debate regarding our choices, because they were our personal choices. I also realized that it allowed the other person time to relax knowing that I was not going to push our thoughts and ideas on them, or accuse them of making poor choices in their own lives. And aside from our girls sharing insider information about Santa Claus being a fictional character with their friends, who were children of my friends, we were able to peacefully co-exist in dance class, at the barn, within Mother's Day-out groups, and the grocery store.

Through our homeschooling adventures, we developed an attitude of flexibility and patience with ourselves and the process, adding curriculums, and adjusting to the girls' different learning styles. We enjoyed special field trips, and personalized cooking or art classes. They were able to commit to projects and activities that they were truly passionate about like music, horses, and dance without the restrictions of a city-school calendar.

We even had our own home-school mascot, the salmon, because we were swimming upstream. We learned some good lessons along the way, and believe me, we didn't always get it right, but we were quick course correctors, and adjusted accordingly when necessary. Year after year.

Our daughters blossomed into radiant human beings, full of love and compassion for others, able to communicate with not only their peers, but, respectfully, with adults. They passed all their mandatory classes, graduated with honors, and learned daily and necessary life lessons along the way. Those same people were watching. And the weirdness was replaced with wonder.

What I noticed over time is that the "whys" got replaced by "hows." Instead of cornering me at a party and demanding, and I am not exaggerating, to know why I thought that home-schooling was a good idea, I am now being cornered and timidly asked, "how?" "How can I do this with my children?" "Will you meet with me so you can share your story and show me how?" "Do you think I am capable?" Instead of demanding to know why we hadn't vaccinated, it's "can you direct me to a pediatrician that will talk to me about an alternate vaccine schedule?" Instead of criticizing our chiropractic model of healthcare, they are asking how it will benefit them, if it will help to prevent a third or fourth attempt at tubes in their children's ears, or if it will correct scoliosis, and sciatica pain. Instead of scoffing at herbal tinctures or whole-food supplements, they are asking for natural remedies and dietary guidelines for Crohn's disease or depression or blood sugar issues. There is a time and a place for drugs and surgery, but these same people are now taking the time to evaluate viable, trusted, proven alternatives before it's too late. The pieces and parts can't be put back, and drugs simply mask the underlying causes, necessary for some, but not most. We are seeing it more and more. The old ways set by society's standard are just not working. Fast is not better. Busy is not best.

There is a different way, in our opinion, a better way. It has worked for us for 30 years, and there's been a plea to share these secrets, so we are. We want to help with the "hows." We want to be a link to truth. We want to present clear solutions, and healing paths to your very own Living Well life. If you want to know more, read on.

Principle 5. Fight or Flight

Imagine you're enjoying a walk in the woods on a beautiful spring day. The sunlight feels warm on your skin after a long, cold winter. As you're taking in the sights, sounds, and smells of a fresh spring forest, you hear a rustling in the brush ahead. You see movement in the brush followed by low-level grunts. Your senses tell you that these are the signs of a freshly un-hibernated, and therefore hungry, bear. Immediately, and without your consent, you feel changes in your body. Changes in your breathing, heart rate, gut, and maybe even bladder come into focus. Your muscles are tense and everything else is now on hold as you must quickly decide what to do next.

How Stress Changes Your Body

These changes in your physiology are but a thumbnail sketch of the changes taking place. Chemically, adrenal glands are now flooding your bloodstream with adrenaline[10] and cortisol[11]. Your digestive and immune systems have officially been put on hold. Sugars and cholesterol are also flooding the bloodstream from their

---

[10] A hormone secreted by the adrenal gland in times of stress that results in increased heart rate and breathing in order to prepare the muscles for exertion.

[11] A hormone produced by the body in times of stress that increases glucose (fuel) for the body by tapping into reserves.

storage areas as the need for additional energy becomes more eminent. You may experience a tunneling of your vision. Your brain laser-focuses on the bear, and shuts out everything non-bear, including immune function, memory, sleep, and sexual function. At that moment, you don't need to fight germs, remember much, sleep, or attract a mate. You just need to survive your encounter with the bear.

This phenomenon is commonly known as the "fight-or- flight response." You may also have heard it referred to as the "stress response." Your instincts will force you to either flee the situation or fight for your life. Either way, your body is engineered to prepare for the task without your conscious input. It's automatic, thankfully. Can you imagine having to remember the sequence necessary to do it on your own? "Ok liver, I'm going to need exactly 400 mg of a sugar/cholesterol mix. Lungs, let's rev breathing up to 60 breaths per minute. I'm gonna need the heart to pump at 100 beats per minute for the next 8 minutes to deliver all that oxygen where it needs to go." No one would be alive to tell the story if that were the case. Our ancestors were much tougher than us -- by necessity. But even they would never have made it if that response was under their conscious control.

The good news is that it isn't.

SYMPATHETIC DOMINANCE

Your body's response to a situation like this is called the "stress response," or, more accurately, "Sympathetic Dominance." Your autonomic nervous system controls the things you don't manage voluntary. It acts, as the name implies, automatically. How do the pupils in your eyes know when to dilate and when to contract? How do stomach juices know when to flow? How do pancreatic enzymes know when to do their thing? Autonomics.

On the other end of the autonomic spectrum are the changes that happen once the danger or stressor has passed. The system is then engineered to "reset" itself. Parasympathetic changes [12] begin to reestablish the normal levels of function. The opposite of fight- or- flight is rest and digest. This is the parasympathetic response. Cardiac changes settle back to resting normal. Digestion, blood sugar levels, sex hormones, and normal breathing are re-established. The immune response is allowed to normalize and we can settle back into business as usual until the next episode is perceived.

I would argue that, by any definition of the word, this automatic response is brilliant. On a cellular level, the body is adapting to its surroundings. That alone would be

---

[12] The parasympathetic part of your nervous system is the part that is in charge of slowing down your heart and breathing rate, and regulating the smooth muscles in your digestive tract.

amazing; but the fact that it is done with split-second timing, with a precision that puts the finest Swiss watch to shame, makes it nothing short of miraculous.

While it is a well-engineered survival mechanism, it is, however, not intended for long-term activation. It works for minutes or maybe even hours, but not for days, weeks, or years. If you maintain this state for too long, it can damage your body. The reason is obvious: chronic elevation of heart rate and sugar levels coupled with chronic immune and digestive suppression are the recipe for disaster and disease. In other words, if you interrupt ease for extended periods of time, you get dis-ease. If it becomes chronic beyond the body's ability to adapt, it becomes full blown disease. The system then kicks in to manage the very predictable secondary responses to the natural response to a chronically stressed life.

Unfortunately, your conscious mind is only part of the equation. Your subconscious mind, however, doesn't filter fact from fiction. This is why scary movies are actually frightening, even when you know they consist of just actors and special effects. It's why goosebumps cover your flesh, why that stone settles in the pit of your stomach, why tears flow, and why your heart pounds in a movie theater. Your subconscious mind is simply taking in information and reacting to it. Immediately. Without thoughts interfering.

It works both ways – positive and negative. Things that make you laugh uncontrollably are as powerful as things that scare the pants off of you. The chemistry of positive reaction is identical to, and just as easy as, eliciting the chemistry of a negative reaction. It's about choosing your stimulus wisely.

Consciously, when you are in a movie theater, you know that what you are seeing is just a movie. Subconsciously, your body doesn't care what your brain knows. It just responds to the stressors you subject it to. This is why music, video games, and other media matter so much to your overall health. They elicit a response over which you have little to no control.

While this may not seem like a big deal in the short term, the long-term consequences can be devastating to your body and mind. Prolonged exposure to these reactions and changes in your physiology lock a feedback loop into the brain that becomes difficult to interrupt and reset. This feedback loop means that heart disease has become a leading cause of death. Chronic immune suppression means that cancer wins.

To make matters worse, our traditional healthcare delivery system offers little – if anything at all – other than attempting to manage this chronic sympathetic overload by throwing chemicals at it. These chemicals, these so-called 'medicines,' are designed to override your natural signals. You need these natural signals to tell you when your homeostasis is out of whack. These chemicals do nothing to correct the underlying problem – they only drown out your body's cries for help.

Statistically speaking, 80% of the disease processes we're currently managing as a nation are a direct result of this normal response to a stressful life[13]. Lifestyle choices drive sickness.

CHEMICALLY ALTERING NATURAL RESPONSE

We've been led to believe that, if we can just lower the numbers, we will have a successful outcome. We have the false belief that we can do this without addressing why the numbers were elevated in the first place. Is your blood pressure too high? Take this pill. Is your heart rate too high? Lower it with this medication. Too much stomach acid? Lower it with this chemical. Trouble fighting infection? Change it with this foreign substance. Feeling blue? Mask it with this magic formula. When the host of adverse effects come from these potions and pills, we have a potion or pill to counteract that. Opioid induced constipation? Take this – it will help.

It's ironic that we tell our children to stay away from drugs, while at the same time we give them drugs.

---

[13] http:www.cdc.gov/chronicdisease/overview/index.htm

"Don't do drugs, Tommy. They're bad. But take this cold medicine for your sniffle." Do you see the contradiction? It borders on outright hypocrisy. And then we act surprised when their boyfriends break up with them or they don't make the football team and they want a pill to fix that problem as well. The mindset of "feel bad = take something" has created an entire nation of drug-addicted, slow-thinking, numb-brained people living something other than their best life.

Your body is smart, but it doesn't differentiate between legal and illegal drugs. Nor should it – what is legal or illegal changes all the time, and drugs are drugs, whether you get them from a doctor or the teenager on the street corner. Your body won't reject one because it is 'illegal' and accept the other.

VITALIZERS:

1. Stress isn't just emotional – it's physical. Be aware of the heightened state of distress that your body is in when you are reacting.

2. Not all stress is bad – some of it is necessary for survival. Understand the response and use it for its purpose and then move on.

3. Chemically altering your body's natural responses will only create more problems. Find natural

solutions to de-escalate stress when the trigger has passed.

NOTES FROM LISA:

Thoughts create reality and focus changes physiology. Stop right now and think about something in your past that was incredible. The birth of a child, marrying the love of your life, the first time you saw the awe-inspiring Grand Canyon or the transparent colors of the Caribbean Sea... anything you remember as magical and transformative... how does that make you feel?

Blessed?
Blissful?
Balanced?

Emotions of joy, happiness, and elation actually begin to energize you and change your body chemistry in ways proven to boost your immune system and relieve stress on your heart! Staying in that place of peace is possible even under the most stressful circumstances!

As an overwhelmed momma of three young daughters, I unintentionally discovered the therapeutic benefits of laughter therapy in a most delightful way! We enjoyed visiting Barnes & Noble with the girls. They loved it and we loved it. It was free entertainment and we enjoyed exploring and selecting books for each of us. On one excursion, we found a book that seemed age appropriate for the girls, and we plopped down in B&N's comfy kid's reading area to see what it was all about. It was called "Junie B Jones & the Stupid Smelly Bus". The girls weren't allowed to use the word "stupid" so they immediately began giggling! I started the first chapter with them, and seriously laughed out loud in the middle of the store with tears rolling down my face! The girls were laughing too. They may have been laughing at me more than at Junie B. We purchased that book and I stalked Barnes and Noble for new releases since 1992 until my collection of this Barbara Park's bestselling series was complete!

Reading these books was very healing for me, and for our young family, but laughter is everywhere that you look... if you're looking! Stop at a local park and watch the children playing; laughter bubbles over in those young, innocent beings; in fact, they laugh more than 400 times per day compared to adults who barely average a measly 15 times per day! Watch a funny movie or silly sitcom (mute the commercials). Encourage your animals to do crazy pet tricks! Look at photos of people laughing. Join a Laughter Club - yup, it's a thing! Just train your brain to laugh easily and laugh a lot.

Apparently the adage, "Laughter is the best medicine" has research to back up the claim. According to some studies[14], a healthy dose of laughter has resulted in physical benefits, such as:

---

[14] See https://www.ncbi.nlm.nih.gov/pubmed/24682001 and http://www.umm.edu/news-and-events/news-releases/2000/laughter-is-good-for-your-heart-according-to-a-new-ummc-study and https://www.omicsonline.org/open-access/effects-of-laughter-therapy-on-anxiety-stress-depression-and-quality-of-life-

- Enhanced oxygen intake resulting in better organ function, lung capacity and cardiovascular efficiency
- Elevated physical and emotional relaxation
- Release of endorphins - the body's happy hormones
- Relief of indigestion and stomach discomfort
- Elimination of pain
- Balanced blood pressure and heart rate
- Brighter, more radiant skin
- Improved mental function, such as alertness, memory, creativity
- Strengthen social bonds and relationships

In a slumpy slump, or feeling overwhelmed?? Count backwards from 10 to 1, and then LAUGH out loud! We were born with the gift of laughter. It's an innate therapy. It lifts our spirits and fills us with joy. It's contagious and unites people. It can help us feel more alive and empowered. It may feel ridiculous at first, but the more you laugh, the easier it will be! Say a prayer of thanks for rebooting your attitude, and allow this pattern interrupt to dramatically increase your vitality, passion and positivity!

---

in-cancer-patients-1948-5956-1000362.php?aid=60533 for more information.

Principle 6. Normal vs. Average vs. Common

When it comes to the concept of what is 'normal' as it relates to health, answers are going to vary. This is true whatever kind of health you are talking about – mental, social, spiritual, or physical. The reason is, I think, because we carelessly assume the words "normal," "common," and "average" are synonyms, when they really aren't.

WHAT IS 'NORMAL' ANYWAY?

Dictionary.com provides us with the following definitions:

NORMAL – NAWR-muhl [adj.]

1. Conforming to the standard or the common type; usual; not abnormal; regular; natural

2. Serving to establish a standard

AVERAGE - AV-er-ij [noun]

1. A quantity, rating, or the like that represents or approximates and arithmatic mean

2. A typical amount, rate, degree, etc.; the norm

COMMON - COM-uhn [adj.]

1. Belonging equally to, or shared alike by two or more or all in question

2. Pertaining or belonging to an entire community, nation, or culture; public

3. Joint; united

4. Widespread, general, ordinary.

Is Jim Normal or Just Common?

Jim has a left hip that aches. He was an athlete in high school. Back in the day, he played three sports, lettered in each, and has the stories and scars to prove it. Now he's 40. A few years ago, he started experiencing occasional stiffness after certain kinds of activity. A few anti-inflammatory pills would solve the problem and he went about his business.

After a while, however, anti-inflammatory pills quit helping him. Ache went to pain, and occasional discomfort went to constant agony. A small limp getting up from a chair became a chronic battle to get from the house to the car. Finally, after some prodding, Jim consented to an appointment with the family doctor.

"Well, Jim," said the doctor. "You are getting older, you know. The Glory Days have taken their toll. This is normal for a man your age. Let's try this medication for a week or so. If they don't help, call me back and we'll go from there. And...so long as you are here, your blood pressure is a little high. I'm going to give you this medication to bring it back down to normal."

The doctor will not bother to find out why one hip bothers Jim and not the other. There is no attempt to discover why Jim's blood pressure is elevated.

All too many times, the Jims of this world settle for this answer and don't ask any questions. They take the advice of well-intended people with fancy degrees, do what they are told by these "authority figures," and take their medicine. It's so common it's a metaphoric cliché – "take your medicine!"

For a time, the medicine may actually squelch the pain enough to make Jim (and all the Jims of the world) think all is well. Until it isn't. Side effects of some kind appear with almost every type of medication. When Jim experiences side effects, he is likely to get more medication to counteract the side effects of the first medication.

Here's some questions Jim should be asking:

- My other hip is the same age. Why doesn't it hurt, too?
- Bob is my age and played on my same high school teams, and his hips are fine. What is the difference between Bob and me?

- Why don't Bob's hips ache if aching hips on a 40-year-old ex-athlete are normal?

- How does the medicine know which hip to go to?

AVERAGE IS A NUMBER: YOU ARE A PERSON

The concept of normal has become synonymous with what is common. Just because something is widespread doesn't mean it is standard. If it were, all 40-year-olds would expect that left hip to flare up no matter what. Common does not mean that it is a mathematical mean. Average is just that, an average of the numbers of each of the subjects measured divided by the number of subjects measured. In other words, if you measured the blood pressure of 100 people, totaled the numbers, and divided the total by 100 you would have the average. 120/80 is an 'average' blood pressure – but very few people have a blood pressure of exactly 120/80. Most people are a little over or under that. See the difference?

No one is exactly like you. They may be similar, but are not the same. Even identical twins can have different responses to the same circumstances. So why would we expect everyone to have the same response to a stimulus? Why would everyone have the same cholesterol count? Understanding the concept of normal body function should reveal the understanding that numbers can and do fluctuate. The reasons why they fluctuate are in many ways more important than that numbers themselves.

Vitalizers:

1. Normal, common, and average are different concepts. Rather than reacting when someone tells you that you are abnormal, or being comforted when someone tells you that what you are experiencing is common, ask yourself what those terms really mean.

2. Check your breaker box!

3. Adjust your routine when you find that your body is not 'normal.' Adjust your diet and exercise routine accordingly. Homeostasis is the ultimate goal.

Notes from Lisa:

In working with people, and managing their health, I've found that one of the most misunderstood and ignored problems concerning what we take into our bodies is endocrine disruptors. What are they? Let's talk about that.

Ultra-simple. Endocrine disruptors are chemicals that we encounter in our daily lives that create toxicity; toxicity, of all types, short circuits our Living Well breaker box.

Toxicity is imbalance.

Toxicity is pain.

Toxicity is stress.

Toxicity is death. (Dramatic, I know, but true.)

Our endocrine system is made up of our body's glands. Each one is integral to life function in its own way. The hypothalamus is the control system, monitoring hormone production from the other glands and how our body uses those hormones. The pituitary is responsible for grown, skin pigmentation, and absorption of water into the blood, and for stimulating other glands. The thyroid manages growth and development. It is in charge of mood stabilization and metabolic function, breathing, heart rate, body temperature, and the central nervous system. The adrenal glands manage cortisol and epinephrine production. The ovaries produce estrogen and balance testosterone and progesterone. The parathyroid glands balance calcium and phosphorus for healthy bones. The pineal gland produces melatonin to help you sleep. The pancreas produces insulin which regulates your blood sugar.

This intricate and well-designed system of glands operates in a delicate balance. The proper function of these organs is vital for life. Can you imagine surviving without any of the functions listed above?

This is why we should care about the chemicals abundant in our drawers, behind our doors, and in our cabinets. These chemicals are endocrine disruptors, blocking, distorting, and destroying the production of the hormones we need to survive.

If you think the things we put on our external bodies won't affect our internal organs, you are wrong. Consider the birth control patch – it is a commonly prescribed endocrine disruptor. It works within seconds and the chemicals in it affect not only the targeted system but everywhere blood flows throughout the body.

Your liver is your blood filter. It goes on high alert to begin the removal of excess hormones so that the rest of your body doesn't become imbalanced. The same holds true for anything we put on topically. Parabens, phthalates, BPA, glycol ethers, and phyto-estrogens are commonly found in body lotion, body spray, shampoo and conditioner, make-up, nail polish, deodorant, sunblock, and perfume. They all matter, and they all have an impact on your health.

So how do you know if you are experiencing toxicity? You may experience migraines, weight gain, challenges with your menstrual cycle, early puberty in girls, high estrogen in baby boys, erectile dysfunction, depression, faulty memory, skin conditions in the form of acne, rashes and eczema, blood sugar disorders, fatigue, compromised immune function, and even cancer.

The good news is that our bodies want to do the right thing. We have control over our choices. We can ensure that we get less toxicity from our environment by managing the things we eat, breathe, and apply. We can consume healthy, organic foods. We can purify our air, drink purified water, and avoid the use of lawn chemicals and pesticides in our homes and gardens. But if we continue to apply toxic products to our skin, we will undo all of the good we've done with those other choices.

Want to do an experiment? List five health challenges that you and your family are experiencing right now. Then, for three weeks, maintain a pristine life style with whole foods, including beets and radishes daily. Use 'green' cleaning products and toxin-free bath, body, and beauty care. Then compare the changes physically, emotionally, and spiritually! Take back control and prepare to be amazed as you begin your Living Well Life!

If you would like a copy of our Living Well list of Toxin-free Alternatives, please contact us through www.thelivingwellcode.com.

Principle 7. He Said, "You Can Eat Anything You Want...Except This."

It seems a bit hard to imagine, but all of the less-than-favorable things we deal with in life today are the result of one bad food choice[15]. The confusion about food, dieting, and the myths that are alleged shortcuts to health and thinness have been devastating to human health.

Fast Food

Growing up as a kid in the '60s and '70s, the era of pre-packaged, processed, and 'fast' foods was just taking hold. Dinner just wasn't dinner unless some shape of colored Jell-O graced the table. Often it was topped with Cool Whip. I enjoyed a steady flow of Coco Krispies, Pop-Tarts, little sugared donuts in a bag, Coca-Cola, unlimited candy, and Dairy Queen on demand. Unfortunately, I have the teeth to prove how these things affect oral health.

---

[15] See Genesis 2:15-17, "The Lord God took the man and put him in the Garden of Eden to work it and take care of it. [16] And the Lord God commanded the man, "You are free to eat from any tree in the garden; [17] but you must not eat from the tree of the knowledge of good and evil, for when you eat from it you will certainly die.""

At that time, sitting still in a classroom setting was not a high priority for me. Consequently, I got to spend a great deal of time in the hallway. By the 4th grade, the guidance counselor and I were on a first name basis. Does this sound familiar? Thankfully, this was a time before psychotropic drugs were used so rampantly in our educational system. I'd have likely been the poster boy for Ritalin.

In retrospect, it seems odd that no one was connecting the dots between how my body was functioning, behaving, and healing to what and how I was eating. Equally importantly, no one was paying attention to how my "processor" was processing what I ate. I suffered chronic athletic injuries throughout Junior High and High School. I was constantly injuring my ankles, knees, and spine. Some of those injuries still revisit me today.

The chemistry that allows food to look and taste a certain way, or to remain on the shelf for extended periods of time, has revolutionized the way we eat. Convenience has replaced nutrition as our primary concern. Cost is a close second. When we can drive up next to a hole in a building, talk into a clown's mouth, and receive a load of something to feed a family of four cheaper than it costs to buy a bag of decent dog food, something is seriously wrong.

Think about it this way: if it will stay on the shelf longer, it will stay in your body longer. The results are constipation, inflammation, and toxicity that contribute to every disease process known to man[16].

WHERE DOES FOOD COME FROM?

Most Americans have little or no connection to the raising, storing, or preparing of the food they eat. We are more concerned about getting to our next commitment. We often drive there while eating something in a wrapper, carton, or Styrofoam shell, washing it all down with a mega-sized toxic drink more chemically related to battery acid than food. We somehow accomplish this while talking or texting on the phone, putting on toxic makeup, and navigating through traffic, all at the same time.

We justify this by saying that it is efficient. We are multi-tasking. Why should we cook when someone else can do it more cheaply? "I don't like to cook!" "I don't have time to cook!" "Can I microwave it?" "Does it have to be refrigerated?" "Can I get that to go?"

According to the U.S. Department of Health and Human Services[17], since the 1970s, the number of fast food restaurants in America has more than doubled.

---

[16] See http://www.medicalnewstoday.com/articles/318630php
[17] https://www.hhs.gov/fitness/resource-center/facts-and-statistics/index.html

Empty calories from sugar and added whole fats constitute a whopping 40% of all calories consumed by children in this country. Adults consume half again as much sodium as the maximum recommended amount. This has led to the obesity crisis in this country, and its relatives: heart disease, diabetes, and chronic joint pain and injury.

Breaking the Fast Food Habit

Let's begin to change things gradually. Unless you are in a full-blown health crisis, small changes are easier to manage, easier to implement, and have the same long-term effects. I like to encourage adding things to your regimen before you start subtracting them.

There is no better way to create craving for something than to tell yourself that you can't have it. For example, there is a huge psychological difference between telling yourself, "I must eliminate all donuts and pastries" and telling yourself, "If I want a donut after I have my morning fruit, I can do that.

Several realities will occur in this instance. If you commit to adding fruit first, your stomach will reward you by feeling full. If you are feeling full, you have less space for donuts. Additionally, the nutrients and natural sugars in an apple will begin to get into your system in ways that your body will love. Donuts don't do that. Most people understand that donuts and pastries have little to no nutritional value, but the convenience and tastiness of donuts spur us to override that knowledge. We can't really imagine Homer Simpson saying, "Mmmmmmm.... apples..." can we?

You've heard the phrase, "An apple a day keeps the doctor away." What if it is true? You'd never hear anyone say "A donut a day keeps the doctor away," would you? But what we know and what we do are not always the same. It's easy not to do the right thing, especially in a society that puts the wrong thing directly in our path.

Your new model is just as simple. Add in good things before you take away the things that are interfering with your ability to lead your best life. You will find that it is naturally easier to take away the bad things once they have been replaced. If you were to keep a food journal, you would see the data. Take a notebook and record what you ate, when you ate it, and how you felt two hours later: physically, mentally, and energetically. Within weeks the enemies will be revealed.

Another thing you'll discover fairly fast is that the closer food is to its natural state, the more beneficial it will be for you to consume. There's an order to this principle: fresh food is best. Then frozen food, then canned or packaged foods. To say it another way, the more processed things are (for shelf life), the less beneficial they will be to consume. It doesn't take clinically controlled, double-blind studies to understand that fresh food, preferably organically grown,[18] will be easier to digest and metabolize than things that have been altered by man.

In the morning, add fruit and a big glass of water. In the afternoons, add the fresh vegetables of your choice between your main meal choice, and more water before any other drinks. In the evenings, do the same thing: add a serving of vegetables and some water. Another "good deal" is to implement portion control. Let your salad be bigger than the pasta or meat serving. Trust me, you'll be glad!

Spoiler alert: this chapter is not meant to be a full-on dieter's dream book. Its intention is to provide a brief introduction to doing things better more often. It isn't about achieving perfection. My hope here is that some of these very basic steps should get things heading in a better direction. Your body will reward you with favorable changes including, but not limited to, better hormone balance, clearer thinking, better sleep, and the need for smaller clothes.

I know what you're saying: "But I can't!" or "I hate broccoli or kale or insert-hated-vegetable-here!" or "I can't live without my Diet Cola in the morning!" I get that restoring and maintaining your health won't be easy. It

---

[18] That is, not saturated in and contaminated with chemicals.

isn't. It's work. My supposition is, though, that, if you're reading this book, you are interested in your health, and ready to take on this project.

Your life, both the quantity and quality of your remaining years, depends on it, whether you recognize it or not. The promise is this: if you keep doing what you've always done, you'll keep getting what you've always gotten.

Keep this in mind: with every bite, we are either moving towards or away from homeostasis. When we "cheat" on our food intake, we not only cheat ourselves, but those who love and depend on us. If you're a parent, know that your kids are watching. The old "do as I say, not as I do" school of parenting always has been and always will be a failure. Your family may grumble as you begin to bring change into the kitchen, but they'll thank you later.

YOU'RE SWEET ENOUGH ALREADY

The subject of sugar deserves its own discussion. In the year 1900, the average American consumed 90 pounds of sugar annually. By 2012 that number had risen to 168 pounds, and it continues to rise. A recent U.S. Department of Agriculture report revealed that more than half of Americans consume a half pound of sugar daily. That's 180 pounds a year![19]

Sugar is the most popular ingredient added to foods in the U.S. It is found in everything from ketchup to soft drinks, peanut butter, cured meats, packaged snacks, cereals, breads, and crackers. These additives are in the form of man-made or 'refined' sugars, mostly from corn. It's a very addictive substance and "getting hooked" is easy.

It seems obvious, but it is worth stating: excess sugar has been linked to the epidemic of obesity in this country. It is tied to the processes that cause or exacerbate many chronic diseases.

Our best advice: eliminate sugar wherever possible. Your body will handle a certain amount of pollution, but, beyond that point, ease of normal function is interrupted. A lack of ease (a dis-ease) over time becomes full-fledged disease.

The answer is not, however, to replace sugar with artificial sweeteners. Unfortunately, as sugar's negative effects have become known to most people, artificial sweeteners have gained popularity as a "healthier" alternative. Nothing could be further from the truth. A quick internet search on this subject will reveal the

---

[19] http://kolpinstitute.org/facts-about-sugar/

dangers of making this switch. Artificial sweeteners are by definition fake. Remember: the closer foods are to their original, natural state, the safer and more beneficial they'll be to consume. Words like "refined," "hydrolyzed," "artificial," and "flavored" are key words to avoid at all costs. When you see these words on the packaging, put the package down.

OFFSETTING THE BEATING

The best way, in my opinion, to offset the things that you cannot control nutritionally is to supplement your diet with foods that either support sufficiency or reduce toxicity. In other words, you should use quality nutrient supplements that regulate your normal cellular function, either by increasing or decreasing certain substances that can interfere with proper function.

Vitamins and other nutrients can replace what's missing from foods. Sometimes what's missing from foods is destroyed in the preparation and/or processing of the foods. Replacing these missing vitamins and nutrients is essential if the body is to function at peak efficiency. Unless you're seeking to address a specific health concern, several supplemental things are not only wise, but necessary if maximum function is to be expected.

Bear in mind that supplements are like any other consumer item. You get what you pay for. Quality can vary between brands. Your body has no trouble telling the difference between good chicken and rancid chicken. It knows the difference between regular coffee and decaf, and it knows the difference between artificial synthetically-derived chemical supplements and those based on organic whole foods. Don't forget: your body is smarter than you are. You just have to be smart enough to know that.

The controversy surrounding vitamins and other herbals is no different than the controversy surrounding anything else. Follow the money. If the pharmaceutical industry funds a study about the worthlessness of vitamins, it would be no different than a study funded by deer to tout the worthlessness of hunting.

Creating nutrient sufficiency is your goal, whether it comes directly from the food you eat or from nutritional supplements. The likelihood of getting all you need from your diet is pretty low. And overdoses are nearly impossible. You'll never hear the evening newscaster say, "And, in other news, the vitamin overdose epidemic takes another life in a local town."

KEEP IT SIMPLE. WHEN SHOPPING FOR VITAMINS AND SUPPLEMENTS, KEEP THESE TIPS IN MIND:

1. Make sure you purchase a quality, whole-food vitamin. Avoid synthetic color, fillers, or sweeteners. The ingredients should all be foods and other natural minerals.

2. Include quality omega 3 fatty acid products. This will usually be in the form of a fish oil product, most often cod, krill, or tuna. For our vegetarian friends, flaxseed oils, avocados, and walnuts will do the trick. Omega 3 fatty acids are like a UPS driver taking other nutrients into your cells. They have significant benefits for cardiovascular, brain, and immune system health.

3. If you live in the Caribbean and wear very little clothing throughout the year, you may not need Vitamin D3. Most of us, however, need this essential nutrient. This little beauty has a variety of benefits, not just as a vitamin, but also for its hormonal and immune properties as well. Vitamin D3 levels are measurable in blood work, so you don't have to guess about your specific needs. Get it checked, and supplement your diet until it is sufficient.

4. Trace minerals are those little micro-nutrients that affect macro-function. Soil quality can be depleted in such a way that even if you are eating nutritious organic fruits and vegetables, these essential nutrients can still be absent from your food.

5. For general health, I recommend magnesium. While its cousin, calcium, is largely responsible for muscular contraction, magnesium supports relaxation. Of everything! It relaxes smooth muscles like your heart and sedates the nerves. It has wonderful anti-inflammatory properties as

well. If your legs or feet are cramping at night, you are likely low in magnesium and need to replace it through supplementation. The only down side to over use of magnesium is a loose bowel. That's why we take milk of magnesia to relieve constipation. If this happens, which may actually be welcome relief for some people, just back off until normalcy returns.

6. To ensure proper and appropriate nutritional supplementation, please visit: **www.yournutritioncode.com**

If you're taking a variety of medications for a variety of secondary conditions, you may want to discuss any contraindications to supplementation with your medical doctor. Don't be too surprised, if they look bewildered or dismayed at your questions. Unless they've gone outside of their traditional training, they may have no awareness, or at least no substantive knowledge, of the data supporting these basic nutritional facts. If they're honest, they'll say so. If they begin their sentences with, "There's no evidence to support...." simply share these two resources below with your providers after you've done your homework:

- https://www.naturalproductsinsider.com/news/2004/09/fda-announces-qualified-health-claim-for-omega-3-f.aspx

- https://jamanetwork.com/journals/JAMA/articlepdf/195039/jsr20001.pdf)

Hi everyone – Lisa here. I know I am jumping into Terry's portion of this chapter, but for good reasons. As a nutritional consultant in our office, I enjoy assisting clients by creating personalized protocols to better their health. We see many types of imbalances in nutrition. My ultimate goal is to provide the tools necessary to rebalance the system, and coach the clients to eat their nutrients in food form rather than by taking supplements. In the initial stages of care, supplements are essential in giving the body the boost that is necessary to set a healthy stage while the client learns or re-learns how to use the grocery store, organic superfoods, and their kitchen to full advantage. Once they are on the right track, they can simplify their supplement schedule and focus on nutrient-dense food choices.

Everyone's health issues are different. Some are dealing with heart issues, digestive issues, skin issues, or autoimmune issues. Some have experienced hormonal disruption, which we talked about in another chapter. Still others have to confront emotional issues. If I were to dive into all those various health concerns, this book would not be the simple guideline that we had envisioned. We will save that for another time, and another book, but I can address in more depth, some important dietary components and why you should consider implementing and integrating them into your life on a daily basis.

Terry already talked about some general supplementation, but let's talk more about food choices, and what we recommend to optimize your body's capacity for foundational health.

Here's the 'whats' and 'whys' of our sun-up to sun-down healing foods list and protocol. I haven't included meals, but we keep them simple with 3/4 of a plate full of organic greens and other organic produce along with 4-6 ounces of high quality, organic protein - eggs, free-range chicken, grass-fed beef, or wild-caught salmon, and quinoa or lentils.

WHAT: **3 stalks of organic celery** juiced with 1 cup of cilantro and 1 cup of water.

WHY: celery helps to regulate the minerals in your body, balancing sodium and potassium which promotes less crystallization throughout joints and ligaments. It also flushes toxins from your body that cause fatigue, lethargy, and inflammation, and alkalizes the system promoting health, and stimulating hydrochloric acid to allow proper digestion of foods. This symbiosis creates less bloating, less pain, and a more comfortable fit in your jeans.

WHAT: **Wild Maine blueberries.**

WHY: incorporate these gems into smoothies, on salads, as a stand-alone snack for vibrant health, glowing skin, and an immune system ready to take on any pathogenic invaders. So what's the big difference between Organic Cultivated Blueberries and Organic Wild Maine Blueberries?! For starters, bigger is not always better. The wild organic blueberry is tiny, and the more plump berries are their cultivated cousins! Both are full of phytonutrients and are considered PowerFoods, both can be organically grown! But it comes down to simple math: the active ingredient that makes these berries so potently nutritious is called anthocyanin, a powerful anti-oxidant. It is found in the skin of the fruit... that vitally important barrier against the natural harsh elements that protect the flesh and prolific seeds on the inside. Cup for cup, the tiny wild berries have twice the skin than the larger berries, therefore they are twice as nutrient-dense. One cup of cultivated blueberries has 6% of the RDA of Vitamin C, and wild blueberries have 15%. Wild blueberries are effective detoxifiers of heavy metals, DDT, viruses, and they are one of the most substantial brain foods on the planet.

And then there is the inherent nature of wild things... wild-caught salmon versus farm-raised, grass-fed free-range beef versus industrial, grain-fed beef. We can talk about those comparisons in at another time, but they are critical to a Living Well life. Wild things, blueberries included, hold innate, survival information. They have adapted to their lives and their conditions in a way that allow them to provide life-giving attributes to those that consume them!

Good: Organic blueberries

Better: Wild blueberries

Best: Organic wild blueberries

WHAT: **Bone Broth**. Read on for all the health benefits, then use the recipe to drink this on a daily basis. I have a confession. I quit coffee. Not on purpose, but because I found something even better. You may not agree with me, and you may decide that this new hot drink is absolutely no replacement for the dark brown, roasted, wake-you-up-with-a-burst-of-caffeine beverage that you habitually drink, but let me share this amazing, old, time-tested, and treasured secret with you. You might decide, like I did, that it's worth including as part of your daily routine.

WHY: I had heard a short blurb on a talk radio station about a little place in NYC called ***Brodo***. It's Italian for 'broth.' A little walk-up window in an old brick building on 1st Avenue at 12th Street serving coffee-style to-go cups brimming with steaming hot bone broth that offer immense nutritional value... protein, minerals, and collagen... enriching your body, mind and spirit. MMMMMMMM mmmm, I was intrigued... and then a bunch of time went by. I didn't think about it again until one of our very wise patients told me that she had started drinking... you guessed it...bone broth! And I was re-intrigued!

I knew that I needed to at least explore this a little bit more. Living in Fairborn, Ohio did not give me access to **Brodo**, and the wonders of their bone broth, but I love to cook, and bake, and experiment in the kitchen, so I was up for the challenge. Our family was pretty clear about how we prepared meals. No shortcuts, no wasted food, and so I began drawing from my heritage (and comparing googled recipes) and went to work.

For the first couple of months, I was discouraged because I couldn't find organic, whole chickens in stock anywhere. And I couldn't special order them from local grocery stores either. Since it is "bone" broth, I needed bones. Healthy, clean bones, with collagen-rich joints. And then just when I was about to give up my quest, a new local grocery chain opened their gleaming new doors! And inside were rows of gorgeous, organic whole chickens! Raising my hands high in the air, I exclaimed, "Hallelujah!!" I purchased the largest one available, which was around 5 1/2 pounds, and headed home.

I experimented with several ways of preparing this magical elixir, and after many attempts, and lots of taste-testing, the best resulting broth came from roasting the chicken, cooling enough to remove the meat. and then adding the carcass, skin, and gizzards to an 8-quart stock pot filled with room temperature reverse osmosis water. The simmering causes the bones and ligaments to release the healing compounds of collagen, proline, silicone, and glutamine that have the power to transform your health. I will attach the complete recipe below, but I want to tell you about all of the incredible benefits that I've noticed over the last several months and also share some of the research that I uncovered about the "side effects" of bone broth, so that you understand the value of this powerful food. I get my spine adjusted on a regular basis, receive nutrition from the foods that I eat and then supplement if necessary, so here you go:

a. Over-all feeling of well-being. Better memory, better sleep due to the glycine, a neurotransmitter, in the bone broth, and high energy maintained throughout the day, no dips or drags in the afternoon.

b. Satiated hunger, improved metabolism, and no more food cravings... for sugar, or salt.

c. Pain in my legs reduced significantly... joints no longer stiff or sounding "crispy". There are many experts touting the benefits of glucosamine to help with joint pain, but guess what? Bone broth has glucosamine, and the chondroitin sulfate in bone broth has been shown to prevent osteoarthritis. Proline is also a player here since it helps to regenerate cartilage and heal joints.

d. I feel physically stronger. The essential building blocks for healthy bones are phosphorus, magnesium and calcium. These nutrients seep into the broth as it simmers and infuse it with these healing components. And the glutamine-rich broth also helps build muscle.

e. Improved immune support. Well, I just got over a little cold, but it was just a little one, that lasted a very short amount of time, and it's the only discomfort that I've had since my bone broth journey began 4 months ago. There are many experts that are calling bone broth a superfood because of its high concentration of minerals such as arginine, necessary for immune function and wound healing. And a Harvard study showed that some people with auto-immune disorders experienced a relief of symptoms when drinking bone broth, with some achieving complete remission. What did your grandmother do for her family when they were sick?? Big ole pot of chicken soup, maybe?? We are all related to some genius women!

f. My digestive system is working better than ever with less discomfort. The proline-rich gelatin in bone broth helps repair a leaky gut, and helps seal up the intestinal lining. This has also been shown to help with food intolerances and sensitivities including cow's milk and gluten.

g. Hormonally, my body feels like a 25-year old's! Happy me! And happy husband! I won't get into the details, but if you want more information about this, you can email me. :)

h. The mirror is making me look younger. Not to be vain, but this was a benefit that I was not expecting at all, but bone broth is a rich source of collagen. Anybody that has purchased a skin care product or has listened to an advertisement knows that it's all about collagen's plumping properties. Your body metabolizes and then uses it to your best advantage when you consume the bone broth internally rather than slathering creams on externally. And my hair and nails are benefitting as well. Stronger, longer, and healthier than they have ever been.

A powerful potion, right?!? Is it enough to convince you to try it for a month???

Here is the recipe that I have been preparing faithfully every 7 days for several years. You not only have the resulting delicious, nutritious broth, but you have fresh roasted, organic chicken that you can keep in the refrigerator, and use as protein snacks, or on salads, or in entrees. Plus I like always having it available for when my grand puppies come to visit. And our youngest grandson, Noble! He likes this chicken as much as the dogs do!

HOW:

Therapeutic Bone Broth

Ingredients

1 whole organic chicken, approximately 5-5 1/2 pounds
Trader Joe's Everyday Seasoning grinder, I love how this enhances the broth's flavor
4 carrots, cut into 3" pieces
1 large onion, or 2 medium, quartered
3 stalks of celery, cut into 3" pieces
4 cloves of garlic, peeled
1 tablespoon black peppercorns
Reverse Osmosis water, or other purified water, to fill stock pot

Preparation: Prepare chicken for roasting by removing gizzards and placing them in a small bowl. Set aside in refrigerator until chicken is roasted. Place the chicken in a parchment paper lined (this will keep the natural cooking juices from splattering in the oven) roasting pan, secure wings with twine and tie up legs. Sprinkle liberally using Trader Joe's Everyday Seasoning grinder or with salt and ground pepper. Roast at 375 degrees for approximately 2-2 1/2 hours, until temperature reaches 170 degrees. Remove from oven. Let cool. Remove meat from carcass and save and refrigerate the meat for another use. Slowly add the carcass, pan juices and any additional bones, or skin from the chicken to an 8-quart stock pot. Add the gizzards and neck from the refrigerator. Add the carrots, celery, onion, garlic and peppercorn to the stockpot. **Add 2 tablespoons of organic apple cider vinegar** which you will not taste, but will help to break down the bones and allow the nutrients to be drawn out. Fill stock pot with room temperature water. Simmer on the lowest temperature for approximately 24 hours. Broth will become golden in color the longer it cooks. Remove bones, and vegetables from broth. Pour and press through a cheese-cloth lined strainer to get smaller pieces. Discard the remaining bones and cooked vegetables. Let the broth cool. Then store in two, 2-quart glass containers in the refrigerator for up to one week, or freeze until later use. To use, bring 12-16 ounces of the broth to a simmer in a small saucepan. Do not microwave. For additional therapeutic support, you can add 1 tablespoon of organic bovine gelatin to the hot broth and stir to dissolve. Drink while warm.

Some additional information:

• The difference between chicken stock and bone broth is simply the amount of time that it simmers. The longer that it is over very low heat, the deeper and richer the flavor becomes, and more nutrient dense as well.

- I do not add salt to the broth. The flavor is enhanced by the peppercorns, and vegetables, and the seasoning that was used on the chicken when it was roasted.

- You can substitute beef bones for the chicken bones. Just make sure they are from clean sourced, grass-fed animals, and roast them first for extra flavor.

- If you cannot get organic bones, do not make bone broth.

- Absolutely NO microwaving. We haven't used a microwave oven for so long that I forget that most people still have them in their homes. Microwaving will reverse the lovely organic process of infusing the broth with all those quality nutrients! It will break it down and change it on a molecular level! And therefore would NOT provide all of the benefits listed in this post! Using a small saucepan to heat it to a simmer is simple and easy!

- This recipe can also be prepared in a slow cooker. I've never used one, so I am not sure about the amount of water that they can hold, but my friend, B.G., uses one to make her broth.

- I've used this as part of my daily consumption, and I've used it in conjunction with juice fasting. Both have provided amazing health benefits with advanced detoxing and cellular cleansing.

- My girls teased me mercilessly about my new habit and my obsession over it until some of their video bloggers, and IG buddies began talking about swinging into their local broth hot spots for a to-go cup as they headed off to start the day! Soooo, maybe their mom isn't crazy after all... maybe she's even a bit of a trend-setter! Now, that's going a little too far, since bone broth has been prepared and consumed by generations upon generations before me. It's just kinda nice to feel validated by your children... and by social media.

WHAT: **Home-grown sprouts.**

WHY: Fresh sprouts are so easy to grow and are vital to our good health and ability to live well. They are high in more than 60 (SIXTY) trace minerals including: iodine to feed the thyroid, iron to build healthy blood, zinc to activate the immune system and repair skin cells, manganese to improve cognitive function, and molybdenum to counteract inflammation and autoimmune disease. In addition to those benefits, they are the best possible source of elevated biotics, which are critical to your body's B12 production. They activate and supercharge your entire system, improving energy levels and reducing depression. This makes any extra effort in growing these little treasures exponentially worth it!

How: You'll need a sprouting jar and some organic seeds. You can find both in the Amazon storefront link at the beginning and end of the book.

WHAT: **Fresh Ginger Root Tea**

WHY: One of the biggest health challenges that we face as a nation is chronic inflammation throughout the body. Each one of us manifests those challenges in different ways, but many times the underlying cause of the dis-ease is inflammation due to bio-burden, and lifestyle choices.

The pathology of inflammation is complex. But let's examine it simply.

Think about what happens when you get a bruise, or twist your ankle, or get a cold. The body instantaneously releases extra fluid and blood to oxygenate the tissue to support the affected area. The immune system sends its fighter cells to ward off infection. This is an important and necessary part of healing. You can see the swelling; you can feel the discomfort and you realize exactly what's happening to your body. It doesn't feel good, but you understand it, and it's temporary.

The challenge arises when this inflammatory condition becomes lingering, persistent, AND internal. You begin having unexplained aches and pains, upset stomach, diarrhea, headaches, blood sugar imbalance, irregular heart function, and you become concerned - rightly so. Internal tissue becomes inflamed due to the same physiological response as a bruised shin. The difference is that because it is hidden away inside of us, we don't see the damage, and it's usually not due to a physical injury.

This modern epidemic of chronic, low-grade inflammation destroys the balance in the body and the tools that are typically used become ineffective in combating the inflammation, and disease and aging are manifested. This process is implicated in a multitude of health issues, such as Multiple Sclerosis, Crohn's Disease, Grave's and Hashimoto disease, Alzheimer's disease, Type II diabetes, many other autoimmune diseases, hormone disruption, cardiovascular malfunction, and susceptibility to bacterial, viral, and fungal infections, among so many others.

The GOOD news is that if we change our lifestyle choices, then we change the outcome. It's a matter of actions and consequences - a simple concept that we used as foundational training for our daughters as they were growing up. It created an environment where Terry and I weren't the bad guys - we were simply the enforcers of the rules. If you choose to be selfish, then a time-out is the result. If you choose to sneak out of the house at midnight, then the result is 3 months without a car, phone, or privileges.

It's the same with our health choices. If we choose to eat that Whopper, then acid reflux, insulin resistance, clogged arteries, and greasy skin are the result. If we choose to eat that baby kale salad with olive oil-roasted beets, carrots and onions, seasoned with rosemary and thyme, and served with a handful of walnuts and wild blueberries, then the result is sustained energy; soft, clear skin; better eye sight; an immune boost; and a restorative night's sleep.

We need to be proactive and make educated choices, so the body can reduce inflammation, reverse the disease process, and revitalize function throughout the entire system. This concept can be your reality.

HOW: Ginger Root Tea: a living well elixir

I use this special recipe integrated into most of the personalized protocols and dietary guidelines that we create for our clients. They experience excellent anti-inflammatory improvement with consistent use. This also becomes a base for combining other energy-tested herbs, like red clover, milk thistle, or rose hips to further enhance the healing response.

Ingredients:

1 large (size of your hand) piece of organic ginger root, peeled
4 quarts of filtered water
Local honey

Preparation:

Cut the ginger root into 1/4 inch slices and add to a pot with 4 quarts of water. Bring to a boil, then turn the heat off and let it steep for 30 minutes. You can have your first cup at this point. Strain some of the liquid, add up to two tablespoons of honey (less if you can) and sip on it for 15 minutes or so. Store the remaining tea in a glass container with the gingerroot pieces in it. Refrigerate. Drink at least 3 cups per day for the most benefit.

WHAT: **Living Well Water.**

WHY: Each and every day we see people in our office that are moderately to severely dehydrated. It shows up on our Zyto testing and it shows up in our energy testing. It shows up in their symptoms... headaches, foggy brain, poor sleep, constipation, aches and pains. I was becoming more and more confused by this because these were people that I knew were drinking the appropriate amount of water per day, so I started to examine this issue more closely.

Just like the earth, we are made up primarily of water. If that water is stagnant then so are our bodies, promoting acidity, disease, and malfunction. Our bodies were designed to drink cold running water from streams, bubbling up from springs that are deep within the ground pulling up salts and minerals along with it. Unfortunately, we no longer have access to that living, vibrant water. This decreases our wellness in significant ways. The water that we drink now has lost its essential nature. The quality is poor, which inhibits our ability to utilize it in our system. As a result, we have become chronically dehydrated as a society.

I found that drinking water in the appropriate amount is not enough. City water is polluted with chemicals - fluoride & chlorine - known to create disturbance in neurological function. Bottled water is manufactured and captured in containers that are full of chemicals that cause toxicity in the body. Well water is a receptacle for run off from pesticides, herbicides and insecticides, or depending on location other chemicals. With these limitations in our water sources, how do we find the best way to use what's available and help our bodies absorb it for proper hydration so that we can function at our peak efficiency?

Recommendations from most medical practitioners to treat dehydration include Pedialyte and Gatorade, but I was astounded and appalled by the list of ingredients in those products. See for yourself how offensive this list is: Pedialyte - Water, Dextrose, Citric Acid, Natural & Artificial Flavor, Potassium Citrate, Salt, Sodium Citrate, Sucralose, Acesulfame Potassium, Zinc Gluconate, and Yellow 6. Let me break that down for you - TWO artificial sweeteners, MSG (a known neurotoxin,) and Yellow 6, which is specifically linked to cancer, hyperactivity, and sleep disturbances in children and adults. You can read more about that by following the footnote if you want to.[20] The whole thing is extremely disturbing. People that use those products are typically the most unwell people. They are the ones that need the BEST ingredients to create a positive healing response in their frail bodies. Yes, it makes me angry. It really does.

So what are the alternatives and how do we hydrate properly to heal, maintain, and enhance our health?

1. We can start by eating foods that have a high-water content, like cucumbers, watermelon, and peppers. 20% of our hydration levels are increased with proper foods.

2. Purify your water with a reverse osmosis system, and avoid plastic storage of any kind. My favorites are listed in the storefront.

---

[20] https://www.isitbadforyou.com/quest.../is-yellow-6-bad-for-you

3. Fortify that water with an infusion of fresh organic lemons, colima sea salt, and honey. Adding 1/4 of a teaspoon of these trace minerals drops that improve energy flow between the cells of the body, help to clear your mind, balance the sodium, potassium and magnesium levels in your body, hydrate your cells for sustained productivity, and increase cell regeneration helping you look and feel younger. It's an excellent addition to your living water.

4. As a guideline, continue to drink 1/2 your body weight in ounces every day.

5. Avoid all products that are artificially sweetened and/or have food dye additives.

These simple steps will help bring life back into your water which will bring life back into you!

If you would like a copy of our Living Well Water recipe, an excellent electrolyte replacement drink, please go to www.thelivingwellcode.com.

WHAT: **Living Well Beauty Chocolates**.

WHY: 1 - 2 ounces per day for deliciously delivered anti-oxidant support along with rice-derivative phytoceramides for radiant skin. Most people understand the importance of protein, fats and carbohydrates for the sustenance of life, but did you know that micronutrients like manganese, copper and zinc are the catalysts that cause the macronutrients to deliver energy and vital function throughout the body?? They are the "coal" that fires up the steam that makes the engine go!! That's YOU!

These micronutrients are also known as Trace Minerals. They are found within the Earth's surface - some deeper than others. God's Earth used to be abundant in these trace minerals and the foods that were grown and harvested were overflowing with nutritional value because these minerals were incredibly bountiful! But the soil has become depleted, and therefore, the foods we eat are depleted, too. We don't need a lot of the micronutrients, but when we are deficient, our systems begin to fail. More and more people are suffering from tremors, hair loss, skin issues, irregular menstrual cycles, prostate disorders, hyperactivity, asthma, or dyslexia, and also lowered resistance to colds and flu, or auto-immune disease. Some people struggle with issues of irritable bowel syndrome or other inflammatory diseases. This is where those micronutrients come in to support and deliver the macronutrients to the immune system, or the neurological system, or the integumentary system to allow for restoration! It's essential! Literally.

Simple and easy! Let's use our foods as they were designed... to sustain us, to energize us, and to provide all the nutritional support that our bodies need. However, if you are concerned about whether your zinc levels are adequate, let us know! We have a non-invasive test to determine if supplementation is right for you!

WHAT: **Chaga Coffee**.

WHY: This brown powder is actually a potent elixir that helps to regulate and balance every system of the body. It is known by a number of different endearing terms, such as "Gift from God", "Mushroom of Immortality", "Diamond of the Forest", and "King of Plants!" Those pretty impressive nicknames were allocated to this nutritionally dense substance because of its ability to attack pathogens and release toxicities. It has been touted for its magical healing ability. Technically a pre-mushroom growth, Chaga Mushroom works to build immunity by revitalizing the white blood cell count so that your body can battle invaders including toxins, viruses, bacteria, as well as unhealthy fungi, and mold. It strengthens the bone marrow, and balances blood platelets. It reduces the aftermath of a "cytokine storm" which is the result of the body overreacting to a pathogen or a toxin. The immune system races to attack the intruder, but at a cost. You can't go to war without incurring battle scars, even if you are victorious. Sometimes those battle injuries include expanding blood vessels, hives, rashes and fever, but with Chaga, the body is better equipped to deal with the die-off from these pathogens.

Chaga is one of the most powerful medicinal tools and overall tonics of the century. The phytochemical elements in Chaga are essential for fighting cancer, regulating blood sugar, boosting the adrenals while balancing the rest of the endocrine system, breaking down and dissolving biofilm (by-product of certain viruses and fungi), and destroying unproductive fungus in the intestinal tract.

Chaga is a superior anti-oxidant containing diverse vitamins and trace minerals including B2, D2, manganese, selenium, zinc, copper, iron, potassium and many more. If you are getting adjusted, and are moderating your food intake, consider introducing it to your diet if you notice excess inflammation throughout your body, shoulder pain, or headaches. It can also help with mineral deficiency, joint pain, fatty, sluggish and stagnant liver issues. Other conditions that Chaga has been known to eradicate include fever, rashes, hives, body fungus, thyroid imbalance, and all neurological symptoms such as tingling, numbness, spasms, twitches and nerve pain. It can even help with body stiffness, foot pain, fluid retention, poor circulation and neuralgia! It is a powerful adaptogen that helps to moderate stress throughout the entire body.

HOW: Add Chaga coffee, chaga cocoa, or chaga powder to your daily routine.

WHAT: **Brazil nuts**

WHY: Add 5 organic brazil nuts to your daily dietary routine! Not only do they taste delicious, but they are nutrient dense, rich in essential proteins and fiber, with an impressive vitamin and mineral package, PLUS they provide 70% of the recommended daily allowance of selenium! SEVENTY PERCENT!! The highest of all foods!

So who cares about selenium??? Your brain and your pineal gland!

Two of the health concerns that we frequently see in our office are depression and sleep-deprivation. Many times these issues are looked at separately, but physiologically speaking they are connected. Research has shown that when people are depressed, they have trouble falling asleep, and then have trouble staying asleep. They wake in the morning feeling just as fatigued as when they went to bed with an added dose of frustration. Their melatonin levels test low on the Zyto Bio-communication device, and they talk about napping a lot. And for those people that aren't sleeping well, they become even more depressed. It's a miserable negative cycle.

But good news!! Selenium is a master mood-booster! It converts to serotonin - the "happy hormone," which then converts to melatonin. All of this allows the pineal gland to do its job effectively by delivering a restful night's sleep! This breaks the sleep/sadness negative cycle!

There are other factors to take into consideration, like overall diet, exercise, prescription medication, stress level, and chemical toxicity within your household. But you have to start somewhere, and by changing these 5 elements of your routine, you have the opportunity to drastically improve those aspects of your health and well-being.

HOW:

1. Eat 4-5 of these organic brazil nuts per day

2. Eliminate toxic products - in, on, and around you - that cause imbalance to every gland in your body, including your pineal gland.

3. Make sure your brain and nervous system are functioning optimally by getting checked by an upper cervical chiropractor.

4. Increase B6 levels with 1 tablespoon of organic blackstrap molasses

5. Bundle up and stand outside, looking at the moon and stars for 5 full minutes before bedtime.

WHAT: **Bitter Apricot kernels**

WHY: They are high in laetrile, an excellent immune system booster. There are claims and research that have proven their effectiveness against cancer cells and tumors. The bitter flavor is produced by the amygdalin, or B17, which is an essential nutrient responsible for targeting abnormal cells and destroying them without affecting normal cells. It is also a powerful liver detoxifier. In this current state of our environment, I am always looking to give my body an effective boost to prevent cellular damage. Cellular damage is an antagonist for serious health issues. An excellent healing agent for the heart, assisting in blood pressure modification, bitter apricot kernels can also help with respiratory issues like asthma and emphysema. It gets better: the existence of naturally-occurring benzaldehyde, a well-known analgesic, and the anti-inflammatory qualities of these little seeds make them a natural solution for arthritis pain. Because laetrile and B17 cannot be patented there are mysterious issues surrounding the disappearance of the cancer research documents, and laetrile was banned in the 1970's. We may not have access to laetrile in the United States any longer, but you can still receive the inherent immune supporting benefits from these bitter apricot kernels in their natural state.

HOW: I take between 3-5 of these kernels per day depending upon the needs of my body. They are most effective eaten on an empty stomach after 3 p.m. The best type to purchase are the organic seeds from the Hunza region of the Pakistani Himalayas. They have the highest concentration of the effective healing compounds from that part of the world.

Just like with apple seeds, there is a small amount of cyanide in each one of the kernels. If you decide they are right for you or your family, be sure to keep them with your other supplements away from young children that may mistake them for a snack food. And like I mentioned in the beginning, this is a controversial subject, so remember to do your own research, talk to your doctor if you feel that is best, and get tested to see if this would be an important element to include in your daily routine.

That is a lot of information, but I encourage you to put these Vitalizing Steps to work for you today, and watch your system transform into a balanced, functional and LIVING WELL body!

Vitalizers:

1. Eat natural, unprocessed foods.
2. Make sure your fruits and vegetables are not contaminated with pesticides.
3. When you eat something, think to yourself: do I want a fast-food burger body, or the body of a fresh, organic peach? You are what you eat – do you really want to resemble what you are putting in your mouth?
4. Start a food journal.

Notes from Lisa:

I have the distinct honor and privilege to work with many amazing women every week. We cover a variety of topics, but typically we are discussing ways to improve health through lifestyle adjustments and adaptations.

We cover a lot of information in our initial appointment, and one of the questions that I ask during their nutritional assessment is whether they are using aspartame or other artificially sweetened products. The conversation usually goes something like this:

Client: "Well, no, I stopped using that years ago."

I follow up by asking if they chew gum.

Client: "Yes, oh, yes, I do chew gum. I always have."

Me: "Do you have a package with you?"

Client: "Yes, would you like a piece?" as they pull the package out of their purse.

Me: "No, no, but let's take a look at the ingredients."

I had four of these conversations just last week, and two the week before, and knew that I needed to share this information. I absolutely, without a shadow of a doubt, know that we, as consumers, are truly trying to make better choices. Gum is a sneaky way for us to literally be poisoning ourselves each and every day, though, and to elevate our health we need to have all the facts.

Since we aren't actually eating gum, we don't usually think about the effects of it on our health. I was a gum chewer. Loved it. Loved the minty fresh breath. Loved chewing it as a deterrent to eating. My brand of choice was Clorets, a sugar-based gum. I thought it sounded superior, healthy even, since it had chlorophyll in it. I chewed it for years, and would buy it by the case instead of a single pack, and stash the box in a convenient upper cabinet in our kitchen. Then, one day, I suddenly began to have stomach pains. Like couldn't stand up straight, doubled-over-the-sink pain. And it scared me. I had been a diet coke drinker for several years before that until I realized that the ingredients were lethal to my health, and I quit. It was difficult to quit. The molecular structure of aspartame is almost identical to cocaine, and it's as addictive, but when I realized that every time I drank it, it was turning to formaldehyde, a substance used to embalm bodies, and methyl alcohol - wood alcohol - a known poison, I knew I needed to break that habit. And, then I became diligent about my ingredient detective work. I read every label and diligently avoided aspartame.

But then this mysterious stomach pain started. I couldn't figure it out. I hadn't done anything different. They were getting worse each day, and more debilitating. And then one day, I happened to glance at my newest Clorets box label as I was grabbing ingredients to make supper. And I stared at it. Still had sugar, but there, 6 ingredients down, was aspartame. They had snuck it into this sugared gum. And it made me so angry!! I immediately threw the box away. And within 24 hours the stomach pain stopped.

Aspartame poisoning doesn't manifest the same way in every person. It's a neurotoxin, so it affects each of us differently. For some, it's stomach pain or headaches. For some, it mimics the symptoms of multiple sclerosis, or lupus. It penetrates the brain, destroys brain cells, and interferes with normal function, like ADHD, and OCD, and for some, it triggers the formation of tumors. There is now a known link between Alzheimer's and aspartame due to methanol toxicity. The list of side effects is long. There are over 90 - yes NINETY - known symptoms and diseases directly related to aspartame toxicity. They are all bad, and they are all avoidable!

Aspartame and artificial sweeteners are not the only reasons to avoid chewing gum. It will also cause gastro-intestinal distress as the parotid glands, or salivary glands, trigger the release of stomach acid and digestive enzymes to break down the food that the body perceives has entered the system. It exacerbates Irritable Bowel Syndrome, bloating and abdominal pain. It can trigger TMJ due to the uneven and overuse of the jaw muscles. In regards to the teeth, the acidic compounds can cause erosion, and the constant pressure may release mercury vapor from existing amalgam (silver) fillings. Mercury is also a neurotoxin, adding even more oxidative stress to our brain.

So, if you are chewing gum, I get it. Let's make it as good as we can by choosing better. One option is Simply Gum, a non-GMO, mostly organic ingredients product with thoughtfully chosen assorted flavors. Each pack even includes tiny pieces of paper to dispose of your gum when you are done with it. If you want to avoid chewing gum all together, but like that fresh breath feeling, try drinking purified water with crushed mint leaves, or Newman's Own organic mints. They also have a nice variety of flavors.

There are so many manufactured products that prevent us from being as good as we can be, and one of those seemingly innocent items is chewing gum. I want to help you choose better so that you can be fully prepared and ready to live a Living Well life. Each decision matters. Honest, it does.

I have a treat for you though. Food can still be fun and indulgent at times. I have memories growing up of how comforting a steaming cup of hot chocolate can be after playing outside on a winter day. One afternoon several years ago, I wanted to replicate that for my grandchildren. However, after I nearly poisoned them with artificially-sweetened Swiss Miss hot chocolate, I decided to create a delicious organic version that I felt happy serving to them after their playful adventures in our snowy wonderland! Here is the recipe that you can proudly and safely share with your family:

The very BEST home-made Hot Chocolate!

2 cups organic powdered sugar
1 cup organic cacao powder
2 1/2 cup organic non-fat dry milk powder
1 teaspoon celtic sea salt
2 teaspoons organic cornstarch
1 Tablespoon organic vanilla extract
Hot water

Combine all dry ingredients in a mixing bowl and whisk together. In a small pot, heat 1 cup of water or milk.

Fill mug halfway up with the mixture and pour in the hot water. Stir to combine. Seal the rest of the mixture in an airtight container to use another time.

Top with fresh whipping cream. Serve with lots of love, and abundance of kisses!

Principle 8. Visualize yourself: Clothing Optional

Just as we must exercise our bodies to keep them fit, we must also exercise our minds. Mental exercises, however, aren't necessarily to boost our mental muscles, but also to relax them. Principle 6 in this book talks about the body's reaction to stress. Since stress starts with perception, we must use the mind to manage stress.

It's interesting, though. What stresses one person may have no effect on another. The person that drives you insane may be perfectly wonderful to someone else. My mother-in-law, for example, is perfectly wonderful. My wife's mother-in-law, however, provokes a completely different set of responses. In other words, nothing is stressful until we decide it is. Our physical bodies just react accordingly.

It's important to realize that thoughts are real things. They actually create changes in your body that cannot be ignored. We could all, in this moment, imagine a scenario or recall a memory that would create tears. We could use this same mental mechanism to create laughter, to make our stomachs rumble, or provoke a melancholic mood. The reason is simple: thoughts are powerful tools that affect body function.

One of my favorite things to do with groups is a guided imagery exercise. It's a remarkable thing for me to observe as I watch the group. They go through a realization that literally changes their physiology in minutes. There are smiles, giggles, frowns, calm faces, and sometimes tears. It's priceless.

It seems logical that you can't achieve a goal that you can't visualize. You have to have a clear picture of where you are going in order to get there. One of the most important goals we all should have is to feel comfortable in our bodies. Insecurity leads to conflict as we try to prove ourselves to others. A strong healthy mind is essential for a strong, healthy body. Focusing on your desired outcomes for healthier mind/body will help to separate you from the insecurities and negatives that may be holding you back currently.

Even though perfection is available in your mind, it may not be a possibility for your body. If we've fallen victim to the expectations created by the airbrushed and retouched images we see in magazines and on-line, our standards may not be in line with reality. Having flawless skin and perfectly shaped bodies and faces simply isn't possible for most of us. But we can all fit the model of perfection that our Creator has made for us as individuals. Maybe you have a perfectly crooked nose, or perfectly wide hips. There is such a thing as the ideal YOU, which is not the same as the ideal anyone else. When we go through the exercise that follows, and I use the word "perfect", it is this ideal YOU to which I refer.

GUIDED IMAGERY EXERCISE

Take a few minutes for this mental exercise. If you're not in a place where you can do this now, make a note to do it at your earliest convenience.

Sit down in a chair with a nice, seated posture. Make sure both feet are firmly on the floor. Close your eyes. Now, in your mind's eye, picture your perfect body. First naked, then clothed.

Imagine your perfect weight. Imagine lean muscle tone and how that would look. In this body, how do your clothes look, fit, and feel?

Imagine all of your joints moving freely and without any pain or restriction. Feel how that feels as you bend and move with strength and flexibility. What would you feed this body? How would you use it?

Imagine unlimited energy, clarity of thought and creativity, abundant joy and happiness. Spend a moment just feeling these things.

Now imagine that your friends and family live this same way. Their bodies are also expressing the same level of perfection, in the same time and space. How would that change your connection to them? Would it change your relationship to and with them? For a moment, feel the changes and joy that would result if each of the people you care about most were expressing this same perfection, if insecurity melted away and we all felt comfortable in our own skin.

Now go beyond your friends and family. Extend the same perfection to everyone in your community. Imagine everyone in your city living in their perfect body and their perfect life. How would things be different? Would it change the dynamics of your community? Would it change the productivity, the joy level, the crime rate? Just imagine waking up every day in this place.

Compare the image of your perfect body to the body you actually have now. If it's significantly different, why is it different? Think back to the point in time where you gave up on having that perfect body. What triggered the surrender to allow the difference? What made you give up?

Now open your eyes.

WHAT IS THE POINT OF THIS EXERCISE?

The purpose of this exercise is to remind you that you have perfection in you. You can see it if you just look. Your mind already has the program, and your body has the capacity to make manifest the perfection you just say. The question is not "Can I?" but rather, "Will I?" The excuses are many and the number of ways to justify them are equally abundant. It may be easier for some than others, but we all have it within us. Our Perfect Creator does not make design flaws, only variation in design. The reality, however, is that you do, by design, possess the tools for perfection.

VITALIZERS:

1. Your physical and mental health and well-being are tied together. Make sure you are aware of this when you take steps to alter any of them.

2. Do visualization exercises like the one described here or ones you can find here: https://www.thelivingwellcode.com/freegift/

3. Take inventory of the media, music, information, and people you allow access to your heart and mind. Things that disrupt your joy and self-worth need to disappear.

4. Try a completely media-free week. You'll rediscover plenty of wonderful things you'd forgotten about.

NOTES FROM LISA:

I am not a scale person, and I am not particularly fond of tape measures. But this is what I know: my pants are getting longer!

Which means they are looser!

Which means that fat is melting away!

I just slipped into my smallest jeans. They are the only pair that I allowed myself to keep during a closet purge awhile back. Because I was hopeful.

And today I am having a little celebratory dancing-with-myself party!! In a sassy little pair of jeans!

Here is the best part of all... because of the Living Well Purification system and a tiny bit of willpower, it only took me 21 days to lose 16 pounds! Jeans that didn't fit three weeks ago... fit me perfectly today!

Physically, my system was supported with whole food supplementation and nutrient dense organic fruits, vegetables, non-gluten grains, organic protein, and healthy fats - and I could eat as much as I wanted of those foundational components! The process was simple, but not always easy. Emotionally, I knew that I needed to break some bad habits, and release a sugar addiction, so with the help of one of our Living Well Transformation specialist, I was able to identify the underlying emotions that were creating these addictive patterns, and break the cycle - I lost weight AND gained the freedom to be the best me ever - with the health and vitality that was waiting for me.

The only reason I am sharing this is because I know there are people who are struggling with their weight right now, which leads to struggling with their health and well-being in every aspect of their lives... physically, mentally, socially, spiritually, and sexually.

Let me be transparent. When I am carrying extra weight, my body is sicker than it should be and working harder than it needs to. Mentally, I feel depressed because I am not taking control over something that I can be in control over. I find it more difficult to be social, which is difficult enough for me, because I feel self-conscious. Spiritually, I know that if I'm abusing food, or being gluttonous, then I am against God's will for my life.

Sexually, well, when I am not feeling particularly sexy, I just want to hide in the dark, or perhaps get a mysterious "headache." "Not tonight" isn't fair to my husband or to me. Sex is an important element of our marriage, and a good sex life helps deal with the everyday stressors of life. It keeps me connected to my husband. It's one of God's gifts to every one of us in a marital relationship!

So: if you could be better, would you choose to be better? I did.

Principle 9. Motion is Life

Surely enough, when we stop moving there will be a funeral. People will gather, nice things will be said, tears will flow, and then we will be lowered into the ground. Or our ashes will be spread. And, not too long after that, everyone in attendance will get on with their lives.

Motion or movement is one of the primary keys to life. Imagine a young, healthy tree. It gently sways in a breeze and bends when the wind blows. Its branches flex and its leaves flutter gracefully. Compare that to a tree whose life force is gone. This specimen, once majestic in life, now bristles and crackles in a moderate breeze. Its rigid branches no longer have the flexibility needed to tolerate the elements. They will split and crash to the ground and decay into the Earth that once supported them in life. No movement equals no life.

Your body is engineered for movement. Your joints are brilliantly constructed for very specific motion and flexibility. To stop moving is against your nature. Movement in a gravity-based environment is essential for the circulation of fluids, nourishment of joints and organs, and oxygenation of tissues. To reduce movement is to accelerate your funeral.

Can there be altered or varying degrees of motion? Can there be injury or other reasons for changes in function? Of course! We all know someone who is so flexible they seem to be able to tie themselves in knots, and someone else who can't even come close to touching their toes, no matter how hard they try.

Just as a willow tree bends in the wind and an oak tree stands strong against it, rustling only the leaves, we all have movement that works best for our particular bodies. Someone who is wheelchair bound may only be able to move their arms. Someone bedridden may only be able to move their heads. The important thing is not the type of movement you do, but that you move in the way you can to the best of your ability.

Not all movement is outwardly obvious. Blood coursing through your veins in rhythm with the beating of your heart; lymph flowing through your body; and air moving through your pulmonary system as your lungs inflate and contract are all easy to take for granted because we don't do them on purpose. They are signs of life, though. These signs of life are evidence of the existence and intelligence of life.

CHILDREN ALWAYS KNOW

Observe children. They inherently know that motion is their nature. They will resist sleep, sitting for prolonged periods, and anything that equates to being sedentary. How long can you imagine a young child sitting at a formal dinner before you have to say, "Stop moving!" "Stop wiggling!" or "Be still!" It is the parent's mantra – and yet it is contrary to the essential nature of children.

Children are naturally more flexible than adults. They run and play and stretch and tumble and appear to be made out of rubber. Babies lay on their backs, grasping their feet and put their toes in their mouths. Now that I am in my 50's, for all the money in the world I couldn't put my toes in my mouth. (Of course, I no longer have the desire to do this, either, but I would like that kind of flexibility.)

These children are in their natural state, listening to their bodies instead of their minds, and doing what instinct tells them to do. Many of us, as adults, listen to our minds – what we think we should do or are expected to do – rather than our bodies. By contrast, gymnasts, martial artists, yogis, and athletes of all sports recognize the importance of proper movement at any age.

What We've Lost as Adults

Compare and contrast what these children and athletes do in comparison to what your average adult does or doesn't do. Many of us avoid movement at all costs. We conserve our energy, saving it for who knows what. We'll circle a retail parking lot innumerable times to find the closest parking place just to avoid a few steps. We even do this at the parking lot at the gym! We'll seek the easy comfort of the escalator over a flight of 15-20 stairs. We'll take a moving sidewalk if that's an option. We can't wait to get from our stagnant cubicle at work to the comfort of our easy chairs. We don't even pretend – we call these chairs "easy chairs" or "lazy boys." The irony is quite revealing – even though we know that movement is life, many are seeking to reduce their movement.

Take this one step further and visit a nursing home. Tired, brittle folks who were once vibrant examples of life, now spend more time in bed than anywhere else. Their frail bodies bristle and crackle with even the simplest movement. The staff does their best to initiate mobility, but they are often met with a mind of resistance. This resistance is exacerbated by the taint of a plethora of medications designed for sedations. These patients would move if they could, but they can't.

What went wrong? Well, for some it is the inevitable process of aging. Poor oxygen levels can make even the simplest of movements exhausting. The loss of balance and brittleness of aged bones makes the fear of falling a real and legitimate threat. Sometimes this is a natural consequence of existing on the Earth for many years. Sometimes it is a result of lifestyle choices made years ago. For some, the mind is willing but the body isn't able. For some, it is the opposite – they can move, but they aren't willing to do so.

No one is asking you to do the impossible. If you can't, you can't. You may be at the point in your life that simply getting out of bed to use the bathroom is exhausting. My point is this: keep doing what you can do. Continue to get out of the bed to use the bathroom, not the other, easier options you may have. Move as much as you can.

I remember seeing a documentary once about a woman who weighed several hundred pounds and could not get out of bed. One day, she decided she was going to make better choices. She wanted to exercise, but she couldn't get out of bed. So she clapped her hands to the rhythm of music. This simple act, to her, was exhausting. But she did it. Again, and again. And soon, she was able to swing her arms. Then she could do more. And soon, she was doing simple exercise videos in her home. She managed to go from morbidly obese and bedridden to healthy and fit.

She will never run a marathon, but she can live her Living Well Life. Sometimes it takes baby steps, and sometimes you will never get beyond baby steps. But don't let that discourage you from taking your baby steps.

If all you can do is clap your hands, then clap your hands. If all you can do is nod your head, then nod your head. Do what you can, and the rest will come in increments.

And remember the dandelion principle – the seeds you spread by your example, both within and without yourself can carry across the world. This woman, who I've never met, inspires me daily when I think things are beyond my reach. And every step of progress I make inspires me to take more steps.

INFORMATION IS POWER - AND HEALTH

In my practice, I have healthy, vibrant seniors and less-than-healthy, vibrant seniors. Actually, we have people of all ages in these two categories. The primary difference between the two groups is information and action. At some point, the healthier group was exposed to information and choices that they acted on. That's it. Blaming our current health status on our genes and ancestors no longer holds water. Yes, it's "different now."

Our understanding of epigenetics has completely changed the way we understand our genetic propensities.

Epigenetics is a field of study which stands for the idea that genes are not sufficient in and of themselves to cause malfunction. Let's say, for example, that you have inherited a gene from your father which predisposes you to high blood pressure or colon cancer. This does not mean that you will automatically get high blood pressure or colon cancer. It means that some outside factor has to act on those genes in order for those genes to express themselves as hypertension or cancer. That may be diet, it may be the exercise you do, it may be how efficient your 'breaker box' is at transmitting signals, or it may be something in the air that you breathe. The presence of the gene is not enough to cause the disease. Something on the outside of the gene must exert influence over the gene.

We may not always have control over what goes into our food supply, air, water. The information we receive is also easily 'polluted' and abundantly available in varying forms (with varying degrees of reliability.)

Maintaining your body and mind is getting to be more challenging now than at any other time in human history. We're the first generation in recent history not expected to live longer than our parents[21]. This shouldn't be. Life expectancy has generally continued to increase. But what kind of life is it? Do we want a bedridden life with no quality, or do we want vibrant, active senior years?

Our choices will make this determination for us. Specifically, our choices to maintain the purity of our food, air, water, and information. It takes effort. It requires action on your part. You need to seek out information and question those who provide you with that information.

---

[21] http://www.webmd.com/children/news/20100409/baby-boomers-may-outlive-their-kids

That means asking your doctor better questions and expecting better answers. Doctors, the government, or the insurance industry are not going to save you. It's on you to seize responsibility for your own health and make it a priority.

WHERE DO I START?

Movement is vital to aging well. The question is not "Will I get older?" but rather, "How well will I get older?"

The answers lie in the choices you're making now. Some regiment of strength and flexibility training is a major factor in the aging process. You don't have to train like an Olympian, but you do need to start somewhere. Here are a few things to consider:

- Can you do a pushup? If so, congratulations! If not, this is a great place to begin. Start from your knees rather than your toes to build some strength. You may need to start from a standing position and use the countertop or the wall as your 'push-off' surface. Build up to doing traditional pushups with all your weight on your palms and toes in sets of 10 or more.

- Squatting deeply, without any additional weight, is a big deal. Can you do it? If so, again congratulations! If you need to hold on to the counter or a chair back, that's okay. It's just important that you do it. Get as deep as possible and stand back up. Ideally, you want your hips to sink to the level of your knees. Do this in sets of 10.

- How quickly can you cover a mile on foot? If the thought of this makes you cringe, and it may, imagine having to walk if your car broke down on a deserted highway. If you needed to get to the bedside of a dying loved one, would you be able to cover the distance? Would you walk or jog? Likely, you'd do both. Rather than waiting for a difficult situation to see what you can do, start doing some training now!

- Pulling your body weight up on a chin-up bar is another great thing to be able to do if you're looking to stave off the aging process. Have you tried recently? This is a tough one. If you can't do it, see if you can just hang from the bar. Increase the length of time that you can hold your own weight hanging from the bar.

- Can you do one jumping jack? One sit up? One crunch? Can you do a single lap around your yard? Whatever you do, start where you are and move forwards. Continue to work towards being better, stronger, and faster.

All of these things can be done for free, in the comfort (or discomfort) of your own home. They require little to no equipment or fancy workout clothes. They are a good place to start if you know you could be doing better.

The side effects aren't just physical, either. You will feel stronger, sexier, and more comfortable looking in the mirror. This will carry over into your mental and emotional health, as well. A quick web search will reveal the science of exercise and its mental health benefits. There's a reason why they call it the "runner's high." There are actual measurable changes in your body chemistry that result from these exercises.

Think about ways you could begin to introduce movement into your daily routine. Could you park farther from the door at work? Could you take 20 minutes of your lunch hour for a walk? Could you begin the day with three pushups/squats/pull-ups/sit-ups and grow from there? Would taking the stairs really be so awful?

If joining a gym or fitness facility is in your budget, now might be the time. Personal training will help insure proper form and reduce the likelihood of injury. As long as you can inhale and exhale, it's never too late to start. A better future awaits!

Vitalizers:

1. Get moving! Whether it is simple isometrics in a chair or a triathlon, move!

2. Information is food for your mind – just as you should be aware of the source of your food, be aware of the source of your information.

3. Make micro-changes that add up. Take the stairs, park away from the door, get up to change the channel on the television set.

NOTES FROM LISA:

I know that I am a healthy woman, reflecting the perfection of my Creator! I *AM* a healthy woman! I am a *healthy* woman! I feel that way! I look that way! My complete blood assessment and urinalysis says so too!

Yet my little blood pressure machine tells me a different story.

I was mystified. Honestly. My body mass index is in the healthy range which means my height-to-weight ratio is appropriate. I eat wholesome, nutritious and mostly organic foods. But my blood pressure has consistently been hovering around 160/110. For those unfamiliar with blood pressure numbers, it means that I am classified as Stage 2 Hypertensive with an increased risk of heart attack, stroke, or kidney damage. I am unimpressed with that. Completely unimpressed. And concerned, which causes my blood pressure to rise...

My dad and my nonna both took blood pressure medication, and even though I am related to them, my lifestyle is very different from theirs. I receive consistent chiropractic care; I choose to eat well with minimal grains and minimal sugar and minimal high-fat animal protein; I don't smoke; I don't take any prescription drugs, or use any street drugs, and only enjoy a glass of wine very occasionally, about once a year. I drink coffee, and I like to dine out, but for the most part, I would say, and I *do* say, that I live a healthy lifestyle.

Except that nasty blood pressure machine mocks me. Beeping and flashing its little heart at me...

So, I have been working on a new equation... new chiropractic adjustment, fresh set of supplements, including adrenal support, chlorophyll, and valerian root, deep breathing, and soothing music to lower my heart rate... and...the specially engineered walking shoes are my new best friend.

I have been walking for 5 days now. Simply walking. In my quiet, comfortable neighborhood. For free. Enjoying the fresh air. I have seen the benefits in just a very short time.

WALKING. It's hard to believe that something so simple could be so effective. I thought I was too busy for this in my life. I thought that eating pure and healthy, receiving chiropractic care, taking proper supplementation, and loving on my family, my friends and my God would be enough.

For two months, I resisted those flat walking shoes, giving those other new choices a chance to make a change. And then each day since Saturday, my blood pressure showed significant reduction! Just from putting on those shoes and walking! Breathing fresh air, and exercising my heart muscle! It is producing what I perceive to be a miracle. I could do it, and I did do it.

This morning my little BP machine sang out the numbers 130/84. No beeping. No flashing.

And I can live well with that.

Principle 10. Rest is Restoration

Guess when your body does the most healing and repair? Yep, when you sleep. In fact, that's the whole purpose of sleep. Recovering with sleep is essential for brains, livers, hearts, lungs, and muscles – the whole shebang. No sleep or poor sleep results in no restoration and recovery or poor restoration and recovery.

For children, especially, sleep is imperative for healthy growth and development as well as for learning. For the rest of us, cognitive function, emotional stability, and physical stamina are all affected by the quality, quantity, and timing of sleep.

How Much Sleep Do You Need?

Those of you that think you can operate on 3-4 hours a night are likely deluding yourselves. Despite what you're thinking, you are not as effective as you could be. Hormone balance, appetite, and metabolic function are directly linked to sleep. Sleep deficiency is correlated with many health challenges, including: obesity, insulin resistance and diabetes, infertility, and immune system malfunction.

So what does that mean? That means that your ability to fight common infections and allergies is compromised. You won't be able to maintain an appropriate body weight or think as clearly or respond as appropriately as you would if you were sleeping properly.

Sleep deficiency can also result in what's known as "microsleep." Microsleep is defined as brief moments of sleep when you would normally be awake. You can't control it, and you might not be aware of it, but it happens. Have you ever driven somewhere and not remembered part of the trip? Have you ever sat through a lecture and not remembered key concepts? Now: imagine your surgeon, lawyer, pilot, mechanic, or electrician experiencing sleep deficiency. That isn't so comforting, and could potentially prove deadly.

So how much sleep is right for you? Does it have to be the 8 hours we hear talked about so much? The answer isn't so simple, and varies from person to person. But it should be enough to promote repair and regeneration. When you are awake, you should feel clear and flexible, and glad to be awake and alive.

For an experiment, try going to bed 30-60 minutes earlier than you usually do. If you have the habit of crashing out in your easy chair for an hour or two, just go to bed instead. There's no shame in going to bed early. You'll thank me, and the ones you care about will thank you for being more even tempered and clearheaded.

Cindy's Story

Cindy came to our practice at the recommendation of a friend. She was in her early 50s and, overall, she was in good health. She had the usual number of complaints about headaches and aches and pains, but nothing major.

I asked her for more specific information. "Tell me how well you sleep at night."

Her eyes rolled back in her head. She revealed that sleep had been a problem for several years. As her natural body chemistry was being radically altered by "the change," she got fitful sleep at best. As a driven and successful business woman, she refused to allow the lack of sleep to affect her ability to perform. To make up for the lack of sleep, she replaced it with her new best friend, caffeine.

She indicated that her diet was generally good. Her energy, focus, and concentration, however, had not been at their peak in years. Her fitness level was decent, but her weight was getting more and more difficult to manage. She had been diagnosed with a low-thyroid condition, but she was reluctant to begin medications that her doctor recommended to treat that diagnosis.

Everything Cindy was experiencing was something that most people seem to accept as part of the 'normal aging process.' We don't have to accept this, however.

Most of us fail to recognize that there is a difference when we take charge of things we can take charge of. Remember the serenity prayer? We should pray for the strength to change the things we can – and this is one of those things.

Our initial evaluation of Cindy, including her structural measurements, revealed significant deviations in both her spinal structural position and her neurological function. There was a misalignment in her upper neck vertebrae which interfered with the nerve signals to her adrenal and thyroid areas.

Within weeks, we were able to address those structural issues. Her nerve signal balance naturally improved as a result. Now, Cindy sleeps a full night, wakes rested and energized, and reports better energy and clarity all day.

And her "normal" headaches? Gone. They are a thing of the past! Turning around a lifetime of spinal neglect can happen surprisingly quickly. Usually it only takes weeks to months. Secondary issues tend to right themselves along with it.

Vitalizers:

1. Establish a consistent bedtime and bedtime routine.

2. Eliminate the evening news from your bedtime routine.

3. Eliminate electronic screens and devices within an hour before bedtime.

4. Make sure your bedding and pillow are properly supportive. If you're not sure if they are, consider whether you experience spine or joint pain in the morning. If so, there is room for improvement. Your bed and pillow should be supporting a nice, straight spine from the center of your head through your hips.

5. If your mind won't quiet enough for sleep, consider journaling your thoughts to empty them out of your head and contain them.

6. Start a small gratitude list or journal. This could just be one or two things which you are thankful for that day. Your mind cannot stay focused on a problem and gratitude at the same time.

NOTES FROM LISA:

Go to sleep!

Did you know that there is a direct correlation between the quality of sleep that you get and your ability to lose weight? Metabolism does not function properly without adequate sleep. The hormones that regulate appetite—Ghrelin, the hunger hormone, and leptin, the satiety hormone—can become imbalanced when you are sleep deprived. One study showed that people who were only permitted to get two-thirds their normal amount of nightly sleep, ate 500 calories more each day compared with those in the study who were able to get a full night's sleep.

Not everyone needs or should get the widely-accepted 8 hours. The amount of sleep for individuals will vary from weekdays to weekends, it will fluctuate with hormonal cycles, and it will change based on stress and external circumstances. It's important to monitor your own personal sleep requirements, energy test the optimum amount, and then honor what your body needs.

Along with weight management, another added bonus of adequate sleep is better sex! Research showed that women who had an additional hour of quality sleep were 14% more available to engage in sexual activity! New mommas, share this information with your husbands; I can almost guarantee he'll take care of the baby so you can get that extra hour!

If you are getting ready for a test or an important presentation at the office, proper amounts of sleep will stimulate your brain. Your overall intellectual performance will increase! AND there is research providing a direct correlation between adequate sleep and improved athletic ability. Those are just a few of the benefits along with improved immune function, healthier skin, balanced emotional health, and lowered risk of inflammatory disease.

Ultimately, if you are doing everything in the daytime to modify and improve your health: exercise, portion control, supplementation, and elimination of inflammatory foods, and you are still struggling to see a change, then assessing your sleep habits should be the next step. Experiment with these simple changes. They will allow your body and mind to be relaxed and comfortable for a healing night's sleep for all of the above-mentioned benefits.

Try this experiment. For a week, do the following:

1. Don't drink any caffeinated beverages after 2:00 p.m.

2. Eat a light evening meal before 6:00 p.m.

3. Exercise before 7:00 p.m.

4. Turn off the television by 8:00 p.m.

5. Follow the Vitalizers listed before the start of this section.

If you are still having trouble falling asleep, or if you are restless, tossing and turning all night, or if you find yourself waking after just a few hours, and unable to get back to sleep, we have several programs available that can help you. All natural, non-addictive supplements may be just what you need to have a restorative, refreshing, and blissful night's sleep!

Conclusion

A few words in closing:

Over the course of reading these pages, you may have experienced a variety of thoughts or emotions. Some you may have liked, and some may have challenged your pre-existing thinking. No apologies, either way. I've discovered over time that I'd rather challenge thoughts and provide what I know to be true and beneficial rather than worry about any temporary discomfort that new feelings or ideas may create.

Some of these ideas and changes will be tougher than others. The fact is that reclaiming your health is work. Plain and simple.

But trust me – you're worth it.

Here's a summary:

1. You are created for a life of health and vitality.
2. Your nervous system runs the show and lives in your spine. Get both checked.
3. Your body is smarter than you. It will always work to your good if you let it, also known as homeostasis.
4. Anything that interferes or over-rides nerve signals will come at a price.

5. What you eat matters. If you can't be perfect in your diet, just do better where you can. Employ the 80/20 principle.

6. Movement is always better than being sedentary.

7. Mind your mind. What you allow to access your brain influences your health and life and general well-being in a huge way.

8. Remember: you come fully equipped.

Know that your choices add up, not just for you but for all of us. Lisa and I wish you all the best in your quest. If we can ever be of service, simply use the contact information on our website: http://livingwellspinecenter.com/

~ Dr. Terry McCoskey

About The Authors

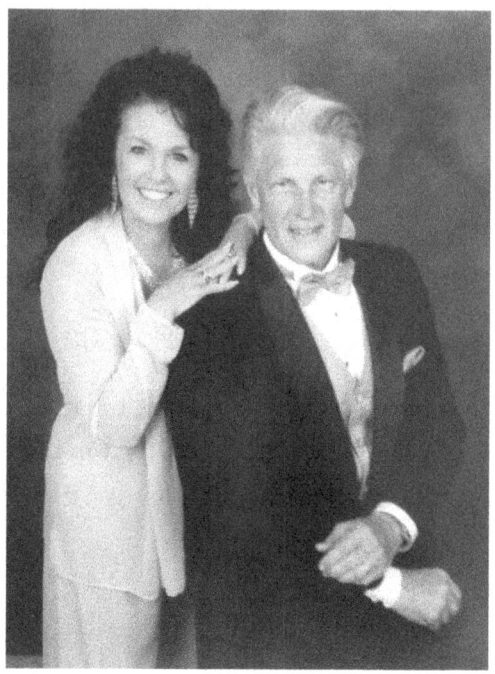

DR. TERRY McCOSKEY has been an upper cervical chiropractor for twenty-eight years in the Dayton, Ohio area, dedicating his life and career to promoting the health of his patients. He has worked to advance the chiropractic profession by serving in a variety of capacities for local, state and national chiropractic associations.

Also committed to community service, Dr. McCoskey is a member and past president of the Fairborn Rotary Club. As a result of the knowledge that he has acquired over his time of service, Dr. McCoskey is becoming widely known as an authority for health and wellness information, and life-style tips. He also serves as a guest lecturer at chiropractic colleges, community organizations and corporations, as well as appearing on local TV and radio. You can tune into his and Dr. Burns' engaging, enlightening, and entertaining podcast: Pair-O-Dox, weekly on iTunes and iHeart radio.

LISA McCOSKEY, CECP is a nutritional consultant, toxin-free lifestyle coach, and Certified Emotion Code Practitioner. She feels that it is imperative to consider the trinity of healing, which centers around our physical, emotional, and spiritual selves. As healing occurs, other areas of our lives are likewise transformed, and we become more congruent with the life that our Creator has planned for us.

You can follow Lisa on Instagram @alivingwelllife, or join her private Facebook group for exclusive hints, tips, and tricks at a Living Well Life. Look for her next book, The Ultimate Guide to A Living Well Life, due to arrive in April of 2018.

Together they have three brilliant and beautiful daughters, Caitlin, Lily & Grace, who are married to their three hard-working and handsome sons-in-law, Andres, Andrew, and Graham, and they delight in the antics of their two exuberant grandsons, Hawk & Noble, as often as possible. They live in small town Ohio with Lisa's white dove, Oliver, where they enjoy spending time with family seeking to serve God in a way that is pleasing to Him, and to fulfill the purpose for which they were created.

Learn more about Dr. Terry McCoskey and Lisa McCoskey at:

https://www.LivingWellSpineCenter.com and https://www.alivingwelllife.com.

Preferred Product Link

Throughout the book, we make reference to many personal healthcare products, as well as unique foods and nutrients. We have created a one-stop shop to make it simple and easy for you to find these same items that we recommend to our patients and clients. They have been tested and used by our family, and are organic and/or toxin-free to enhance your overall health and well-being.

Please follow this link to access our preferred products: https://www.amazon.com/shop/alivingwelllife

WILL YOU DO US A FAVOR?

If you enjoyed this book or found it useful we'd be very grateful if you'd post a short review on Amazon. Your support really does make a difference, and we read all the reviews personally so we can get your feedback and make this book even better.

Thanks again for your support!

Dr. Terry McCoskey and Lisa McCoskey